Seriously
and
Fearlessly

How to THRIVE
in the Massage Therapy
BUSINESS

Suzanne Eccher

Seriously and Fearlessly: How to Thrive in the Massage Therapy Business
Published by Colorow Press
Littleton, CO

ISBN: 978-1-7325297-0-0
HEA014000 HEALTH & FITNESS / Massage & Reflexology

Cover design by Andrea Costantine
Interior design by Victoria Wolf

QUANTITY PURCHASES: Massage therapy schools, companies, professional groups, clubs, and other organizations may qualify for special terms when ordering quantities of this title. For information, email info@colorowpress.com.

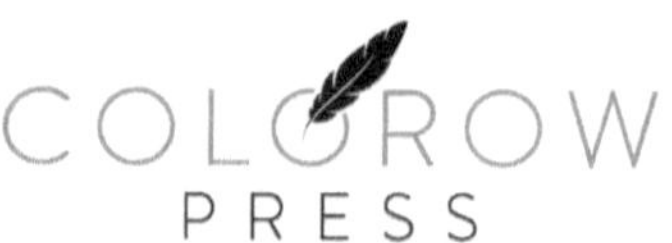

dedication

Margaret A. Olson, my mother, who told me I would be
a great massage therapist and showed me the meaning
of perseverance and how to help others.

My husband, Mike, who has always supported
my passion and business

My daughters, Madeline and Rachael, for sacrificing my
full attention while growing in my adulthood

My Goddesses Tobi Titchener, Charmaine Stattman, Deborah
Peter, Marie Hahn and Lesley VanDersarl who I have grown
with and continue to support me with my mission

Robert Raymond, Vanessa Raymond, Shari Mitteco and
Mike Libercci my Achieve Systems leadership team who
see the vision of integrating all fitness, health and
wellness practitioners across the globe

table of contents

My Story

How the industry has changed

How to be careful what you ask for from the Universe

Snapping Out of It and Getting Started

How putting off going on your own can hurt your development

Change how you look at things the way they are and creating something better

Manifesting Your Future

How to transition your mindset, your actions and instilling your power to change

How you can honor what YOU want to provide

Have No Fear

Be in business for yourself but not by yourself and how to gain confidence

Why you deserve to be paid one hundred percent of your fees

Matching Your Passion With Reality

Does your passion match the client's needs or are you just following a routine

How to create your own income path and avoid the voices out there

You're A Professional

Discovering your spiritual journey as a massage therapist and body worker

Why continuing education and knowing anatomy is vital to our industry

preface

WHILE IN THE MASSAGE THERAPY industry for twenty-three years, I was always looking forward to the day when massage would be well known by the majority of the population and the day when most people would have experienced it. What I know now is that while this came true, it has come at a price for the massage therapist. The independent practitioner is failing in our industry. As we approach 2020, great high-quality massage schools are closing across the nation because they have continued to lower their standards to increase enrollment in reaction to schools that have lowballed tuition rates for incoming students. As a result, the quality of education in our industry has slowly declined as the demand for a fifty-minute massage has become prevalent at most corporate-owned chain massage stores. Schools are conforming their programs to meet the demand of this the high-paced therapist. This has lowered the standard of expectations of the employer, school, and clinics that employ a massage therapist. Massage therapists will tell you that they are frustrated with the amount they earn when working as a massage therapist employee and subcontractor. The independent therapist would also tell you he or she is frustrated because of insufficient earnings while working as a sole proprietor. Seasoned therapists would tell you they are frustrated by this and witness their bodies breaking down, forcing them to come up with another income-generating plan because their earnings didn't generate sustainable income.

What I have observed is that massage therapists generally have no forward thinking about making more money during their careers to set themselves up for retirement. Some have good saving habits, but since we live in an economy where the value of the dollar declines over time, we are mostly working in the moment, and most therapists do not have guidance about saving. What's unsettling is how much the spa industry is capitalizing on our industry. In 2017, the US spa industry reported revenue of $17.5 billion.[1] The spa industry made one billion more revenue than the independent massage-provider industry. While the spa industry often provides more amenities than what an independent massage therapy owner can provide, the spa industry does know how to establish its own pricing because of creating exhilarating surroundings. According to the American Massage Therapy Association in its annual industry fact sheet[2] research shows that US massage therapy was a sixteen billion industry in 2017. In 2016, the average annual gross income for a US massage therapist (including tips) was estimated to be $25,539, and the average amount of time worked each week was 19.5 hours, which calculates to about $2,185 per month. In most parts of the country, that is just enough to pay personal expenses and not enough to pay any business rental or operating costs. According to this

------

[1]https://www.statista.com/statistics/200130/us-spa-industry-revenues/
[2]https://www.amtamassage.org/infocenter/economic_Industry-fact-sheet.html?src=navdropdown

research, forty-two percent of massage therapists say they would like to work more hours of providing massages than they currently do, and fifty percent of massage therapists also earn income working in another profession. The only one establishing pricing is the independent massage therapist, and pricing is as low as forty-five dollars per hour and as high as $120 per hour.

The big-box chain stores establish their pricing to provide affordable massage with membership pricing, but this is a terrible disadvantage to their in-house massage therapist. The average wages for big-box massage therapists is $17.23 per hour, less than that of some receptionists since the top ten percent of people in that job category earn $18.16 per hour. This is a heartbreaking reality, and I was frustrated that therapists felt they could not make it on their own, and that they had to work for large corporate-owned big-box massage stores because they felt they couldn't compete with the corporate model. I first heard this in 2014 from a young lady in my massage continuing education class at the 2014 AMTA National Convention in Denver, Colorado. I was so shaken by this that it never left my subconscious. Even when the standard rate for massage was sixty dollars per hour, therapists were making sixty to seventy percent more of a percentage of that rate, more than the twenty-five to fifty percent that they are today. Why is this acceptable? To me, it is not acceptable. I asked around and did research, and no leaders in the industry were stepping up to make change. The only change we had been making was on our own. However, where did that leave the massage therapist who also needs to be earning more income but doesn't know how to implement a change? Until now there has been no collective effort to help change the current standard in the massage industry.

I was introduced to my current business partner, who had a solution for massage therapists, one that's incredible. The profitable business model used in businesses is not being used by the majority of health and wellness professionals. Massage schools don't teach it or even by mentors and coaches in the massage industry. My vision is to change this, and we are on our way to creating a cultural change in the industry of massage therapy. We will double and triple those income numbers, so that massage therapists can plan their future or stay in the industry much longer than ever before. I was given the opportunity to show how it could be done differently, and I could no longer sit on the sidelines and watch talented therapists leave their practices because they couldn't make ends meet. Moreover, I couldn't watch them continue to fail. I nearly left the profession three times in my twenty-three years, but now I no longer have to worry about it since we now have solutions. The current, and old-fashioned, way of business in massage therapy is about to change for those who want to create a solid financial future.

This book is to tell my story of the years of struggle I had before I found a successful business in massage therapy. We all do things differently, but the fact is that if you want a real, profitable business in massage therapy, you have to think like a businessperson. Anyone can learn it, and now we are teaching it. This business model is for the new entrepreneur who has big dreams and wants big things in life. And it is also for the massage business owner who has the desire to make a lot of money for his or her charity, family, or cause and also has the desire to have financial freedom. We have the ability to capitalize on a very lucrative industry; let's find how you can find a way to do that and stay in it for life if you want to. This book is also for the student out of school who wants to learn what to expect in establishing his or her own business. This information gives that student answers to a lot of common questions with solutions that enable a person to last as a massage professional.

Some may not agree with what I have to share, but this comes from the heart, and I share it because I love the massage industry. I want to protect it and increase the integrity of what we offer. This includes taking care of yourself—spiritually, physically, mentally, and financially. We are so lucky! Only in this healing profession do therapists get to experience the client's epiphanies, transformation, actualization of self-love, self-acceptance, complete joy, serotonin bursts, smiling faces, and the utmost appreciation in repeat visits. I find this the most rewarding career on the planet (parenthood tops it but is not a money-making career). I want everyone to have a chance.

In Love, Blessings, and Light,
Suzanne Eccher, LMT and practice
building specialist with
Massage Practice Building, LLC

my story

WHEN I WENT TO MASSAGE THERAPY school, I didn't know massage therapy would be a lifelong career. I found so much passion in the work that I couldn't imagine myself doing anything else. What started as a skill and art became a calling to serve. To truly make a difference in helping people feel better, I have to have passion, passion to help, passion to serve, and passion to make the connection with my client and use what tools I have to help that client. I am a person who enjoys being in the present moment and relishes experiences, and that is what makes me a skilled therapist. I'm always listening, feeling, and knowing what I need to do because I'm tuned into a client's body, and it tells me what it needs. I spent years being in the moment until I realized that I also was keeping my business in the moment and not striving to reach my absolute best. What I thought working for myself was about—doing what I wanted and working when I want and being successful—was a dream and not a reality because I was living month to month with my focus on making rent and paying a few bills. I definitely was doing what I wanted and working when I wanted, but I really wasn't financially successful. Being successful in massage therapy at the time for me was getting any clients. Getting clients was hard in 1995, I couldn't convey to everyone enough how much massage therapy could help in preventing disease, managing pain, incorporating a healthy lifestyle, and taking care of the body. Industry research was being done, but it wasn't enough yet. We were pounding the pavement, still trying to get chiropractors on board, let alone doctors. Now we are in a place of greater awareness because of the popularity of massage therapy and the many years of research that have brought other caregivers on board with us. It's refreshing to know that today most everyone knows about massage therapy or has heard of it, but it remained harder than ever for me to make ends meet as a sole practitioner.

Being present in my work and staying in the moment was good, but I wasn't making the income I needed to survive. Taking my level of passion for helping others into the business world was extremely difficult since, even though I had business experience, I couldn't connect the two worlds. People like me who do best being in the present are not the ideal candidates to build a business, or so I thought. With this mind-set, I thought of myself not as a manager or planner, but as a helper. Focusing on my passion was much easier for creating things in bodywork. Creating myself as a business owner took a shift in my mind-set. This therapeutic profession allowed me to grow as a person—as I learned how to enable people to heal themselves—through the work of massage therapy. Through it I have learned my limits and boundaries, what to say and what not to say, how to deal with my emotions as they come up, and how to discern if the emotions are mine or my client's. I have discovered my style and how to help people in the process. It took a lot of years and confidence in how

I ran my business, I just needed partners to help me grow. Most of all, perseverance was the key to my success. I had some tough years of doubting myself, my skills, rates, equipment, and attempting to stay away from selling product.

Most importantly, I thought at the time, "Why is it working for everyone else and not me?" As I found out later, it wasn't easy for them either. What was the alternative? Getting another job, going back to school, or quitting this profession and doing something else that was not going to make me happy. I just loved what I did as a massage therapist to let it go. I had to figure it out. I was terrible at marketing. I looked online for tips and how to market, but I found the processes recommended were not easy to accomplish for me. One online site was about making lists and following plans that didn't work for me. Instead, I needed action—not just in business but also in taking care of myself first, conquering the obstacles second, and never giving up.

Why did I go out on my own? In 1995, we only had two other choices at the time, work for a chiropractor or work for a personal injury clinic. My goal in going to school was to have my own schedule and clients. I was drawn to continuing to do massage even if it was completely part time or, as the IRS calls it, work as "a hobby." I had part-time rent spaces to share, and I was only making rent and a little cash here and there. Even though this was difficult financially, I made it a priority to keep my hands in it and to keep my brain and body active. This kept my skills sharp and body in rhythm. I didn't have an extensive network to tap into, and at the time online resources did not exist. I did what I could to get new clients, offering my current clients referral programs, but it rarely worked for me since my current clients had already referred all the people they knew. Taking certification programs was essential to expanding my skills and helping my clients feel better and keep coming back. Some colleagues had their practice take off quickly. Years later I realized I worried more about what I wasn't doing instead of taking action on what I needed to do as a business.

My client base remained small because that's what I asked for. The universe listens well, and I feared having too many clients, so I got what I asked for. The generous clients could not come often enough and I didn't give them the programs they needed. I had a part-time practice with part-time rent when I had to leave my space because of life changes at home. I could no longer afford it, and I moved across town. Unfortunately, my clients did not follow me to my next location. I was asking for clients, but I wasn't being specific about what kind of client I was looking for. What was I looking for? I was focused on having enough money instead of attracting the right client.

I questioned myself all the time. Was this right? Did other people have problems with this? I didn't know it then, but I was stuck because of me, I didn't have the support to stop doubting myself. It changed when I found a focus or a niche that I was passionate about, and I worked in a different way than before. That was because I was ignited by the possibility and the responsibility of letting a specific population know that I had something to offer. As I do that today, it still brings me people outside my niche. I lead with my niche, and others follow. Since I had to leave my part-time office space, I moved my practice to my home. I had a great setup; the only drawback was I had stairs that led to my treatment room. This wasn't ideal since I didn't want to appear unprofessional and not inclusive for all clients, but it's what I had to do at the time.

I had to make a certain level of money after I became a vender for a multilevel marketing (MLM) company. With that company, I was foolishly spending more than what I earned and spending too much time trying to figure out how much I had to sell and buy to make quotas to earn money back. Massage therapists are a prime target for health-product sales with an MLM model. An MLM involves a tiered system of earning income by selling products. In involving myself in MLM, I limited my niche market since I was distracted from what I love to do— massage! Once I got refocused, I saw the repeat clients every week and every month out of my home, and I definitely was enjoying this change. I got a lot done at home. Laundry and household chores became easy to accomplish. I was always home for my children, which was important, but I could have had more options if I had planned better. I looked back and realized I only gained a few clients over two years' time. I knew that advertising in newspapers or magazines for a home practice was complicated; I wasn't comfortable advertising my location, and people generally wanted to know about a business through researching an address. But I needed more clients, now! I couldn't grow because I had limited myself by creating a small environment that had no growth potential. I was right back to giving myself a situation that couldn't provide me with any growth in my practice. I again got what I asked for—a limited practice.

Fortunately, through my MLM networking events, I met a nurse who worked at a local hospital that was looking for someone in my niche market of prenatal and postpartum massage to offer massage at her hospital. I thought this was it, a better source of supplemental income. They had thirty-eight patient rooms. This was exciting! I would be so busy that I would hope to hire other therapists to work with me. These ideas were not based in reality since hospitals at that time weren't familiar with massage services as much as they are today. The nurses I worked with didn't know how to tell the patients about massage and its benefits. It was a few years before most of them got on board. Once they started to, I thought it would begin to grow quickly. I figured I could hire someone to handle my on-call hours, and I could have a room to do chair massage for nurses and have a table for staff. Unfortunately, the administration would not allow it. Years later what it came down to is that my client base from my practice was going to be my best income source. I had to get my practice out of my house; I wasn't putting myself out there. Essentially, I didn't want to be discovered. I needed to find my success with another office-share situation, but this time it needed to be a full-time room. I searched the area around the hospital, but it was too pricey. I couldn't afford rent on my own. I met someone who was starting a partnership center with another practitioner. They had a small space for me to rent. I was a renter for the first few years, and then they asked me to enter a partnership with them and expand into a space that would provide an opportunity for growth, adding four additional rooms with other types of practitioners in mind. Finally, it seemed I would have another source of income to tap into. Unfortunately, there was no plan to do this. When we moved, we had trouble finding renters at first. We had to carry the rent for a few months while the economy tanked in 2008. Not only were we carrying rent for other rooms, but we were also losing clients because of the recession. We didn't have the infrastructure or the support to sustain the large center we had planned. Over time we discovered, too, that our goals were becoming less in line with one another, and when the lease was up, we severed the partnership, which created disharmony and bad morale for our renters. One of my partners and I moved into a new space with two of our renters, creating an equal-share environment. At that point, it was time to try something to seriously recreate my client base. I tried a new start-up networking group, and it failed. Instead, I thought I would make the commitment to go around to medical offices, introduce myself, and give them a quick blurb about what I did, hoping the connection took place for them and waiting for the phone to ring. What was I thinking? I'm an intro-vert! I wasn't going to do that; I never had the guts and would never make the time to do it. Talking to the gatekeeper—a receptionist or office manager—wasn't going to get me to a source for referrals. So I was right back where I started.

I needed people who wanted to help me and learn from me, the professional. That's how I would have the best results. I didn't have the business mar-keting and planning skills to be successful. My acu-puncturist told me to try networking again. I need-ed people who wanted to help me and their client have the best results. I joined a networking group where the process of giving was equal to receiving. In this group, my income grew sixty-five percent be-cause I was in front of people and actively meeting with them to find out how we could work together. We established relationships with one another to do business together. I resisted the networking concept at first because it was difficult to have the energy for it. However, what I discovered was that this became my marketing plan. In lieu of paying for advertising, I invested in my business through networking, which—little did I know—gave me an investment in myself. I found people who validated my work and gave me business. We built relationships that—because we knew one another well—turned into a win-win for us. I also became the public speaker I am today because I had to learn how to give speeches in order to participate in a system that worked. And I took a chance on a group of people that to this day support my business.

The massage industry facts show how upside down we are in having success. Those who have already reached their point of satisfaction in income are driven and work to their heart's content until they are burned out or injured. Being in the moment, they may not have a backup plan or be able to retire when they want to, as opposed to when they have to because of bodily burnout. In general, they have a second source of income to support them, or they live minimally and are OK with that. The statistics in our industry today support the fact that we need change in how we think about building a business. In 2008, the average annual income (including tips) for a massage therapist who provided fifteen hours of massage per week was $31,500. Moreover, ninety-six percent of that market was sole practitioners. In 2016, the numbers had dwindled so that the average annual income (including tips) for a massage therapist who provided 19.5 hours of massage per week earned $26,216, and fifty-eight percent of the market was sole practitioners. Sole practitioners are struggling to make ends meet, let alone being able to stay in business for themselves, and they are dominated by a market in which ownership is not in the hands of sole practitioners.

My mission is to change our industry back to being dominated by massage therapist-owned enterprises. I want to help all healers and bodyworkers enjoy their work and still make the income they need to have the ability to retire whenever they want to and not when their bodies give out. If some massage therapists are in a place in their career where they have to quit, I want them to stop and think about what they can to do to continue in their careers, careers in which their passions are fulfilled. You can still make an impact after suffering an injury, and you can still make life changes to create a financial future. Once you are touched and blessed to be a healer, it's hard to turn away. There are hundreds of opportunities to continue with it and to sustain whatever lifestyle suits you. I believe in everyone's ability to stay in the world of health and healing. It's up to all of us to make a change in how we do business. It is possible to create it for yourself; let's capture your inner CEO.

snapping out of it and getting started

HAVING EMPLOYEES IS A FINANCIAL deterrent for most therapists since the responsibilities are higher due to providing health care and other benefits to employees. You will spend more to hire someone, but if your business model provides a great deal of profit, you will have no problem covering those costs with the right guidance. It's essential that you hire out bookkeeping, accounting services, healthcare brokering, and financial guidance. This team will help you plan for the unexpected, and you will have better success as a business.

How long will it take you to make the leap to create your own massage therapy practice/business? Are you genuinely comfortable selling for someone else, or would you rather sell for yourself? Some corporate massage chains offer commissions to massage therapists based on the number of memberships to their business that are sold. The model works financially because the employer can significantly reduce the amount paid to a therapist based on insufficient sales performance. Did we get to learn how to sell memberships in massage school? *No.* It's OK if consumers decide to buy into this, as mentioned before, because it's better than a person not getting a massage at all, and we can be guaranteed that eventually some of the chain's customers will learn they need more and will seek out an independent practitioner to help them with their goals. So as you embrace the existence of this model, it *will* help you build your private practice, as you will likely get clients from it as long as you offer more and your business is visible. It's a model that isn't successful even though it appears to be. It's a numbers game of consumer turnover and places opening and closing that is not widely published, and, again, this is OK! Some of us know we can't be part of this type of model, and those who do—we want to support you too. To start your business right, we recommend Massage Practice Building (MPB) as your best solution, strategic and immediate, for success with an income-earning-based program. As you start on your own you will learn so much more about the direction of your path as an excellent therapist. In other words, the sooner you start, the better off you will be in establishing yourself as an independent professional business owner. Some started with clear goals of working for themselves, but the process of attending school is so intense and overwhelming that plans can change, especially when they learn the work involved in getting started or more importantly are not provided enough information about it. Schools don't make the time to teach longevity in a massage therapy career, and therefore you are left to either struggle or succeed. Success is less likely since, as noted before, the average income reported by therapists nationwide in 2016, was $25,539. That is quite disgraceful. We need to change that. Never let any advice affect you that delays your goal to establish yourself as an independent professional practitioner. If you need immediate income, there are better strategies you can learn with

MPB that will set you up to earn money faster and create anything you want in a massage therapy business or wellness center.

Every business in massage therapy must use a profit-seeking model. This can be accomplished in many ways. Selling outside product that helps your clients is one strategy, but most importantly you must create a model that sells more than just product. You must sell what a healthy lifestyle is for mind, body, and spirit. Selling a lifestyle that prevents health problems is what people need, and they are seeking it. Medical communities have their place in health care, but what people need, as we know, is to not rely solely on a medical model. Taking charge of their health is what they are looking for, and they are seeking complete information on what they need to do to prevent disease and illness. Creating your business to strategically provide wellness will give them more of what they need. Regardless of whether you are a sole practitioner and plan to remain independent or are hiring others, this is where you need to be regarding future success. If we capitalize on what we know about what benefits the human body—a daily practice that focuses on exercise, self-care, nutrition, and hydration health—we will be successful, guaranteed. In some cities, we are in a great place—where the medical community has accepted the benefits of complete prevention of disease, including massage therapy. It's up to us to take a more active role as providers, equal to that of doctors, chiropractors, acupuncturists, and naturopaths. If your business is located in an area that is less progressive in adopting massage therapy as a part of health and prevention of illness, it is even more important that you educate the community about their options in how massage therapy can help them.

A strategy of growing a massage business or wellness center where you will hire employees—providing them the education to sell more programs (not packages) and where they become the service provider under your business name—is likely to be great for your growth. Select employees based on your mutually aligned goals for what quality care is. Massage therapists who aren't motivated by guiding people through a health journey will not be good candidate to hire. Providing them an opportunity to learn how increasable the accountability is may change this for them. They were likely taught to deliver a fifty-minute massage and haven't learned the possibilities we know can impact a client's life. How do you get them to be an asset to your business? You teach them how. Create an internship to guide them and coach them. In our industry, what I don't recommend is subcontracting. Subcontracting workers legally and ethically has blurred lines and will only be shown to be a success or failure based on the subcontracted therapist you think you can trust. Ideally, you would be better off renting space to therapists and other practitioners if you don't have a profit-building model created with the ability to hire. You must be great at attracting new business to have success in this situation.

What is not understood by those who hire massage therapists—unless they are massage therapists—is that clients come and go. The client will either like them or not. You can never successfully hire someone and control how it will play out; you just can't. The ideal massage therapist you hire must be someone who would never want to own his or her own business or manage a business or practice. Such therapists know their limitations in that capacity and just want to help the client. That is great! As an employer, however, you are going to have to give them something more than a wage to retain them as employees. Overall, what you need is the best strategy to hire. What can you offer a massage therapist to make that therapist truly happy and want to stay? Often you must show you are happy he or she has chosen you for employment. This can be done with employee events and celebrations, and that can definitely be helpful, but ultimately it comes down to the power of the dollar. If you have great programs set up where the client is enrolled in a monthly service or invests in other income-generating products and services, and your employee has met the standard you expect to be delivered, you can expect to make consistent income through what you offer all clients. If the therapist has proven they are a good fit for your business allow them to capture a portion of the profits as an incentive payment to continue driving profits to your clinic.

Having different levels of requirements and qualifications of your therapists is a great strategy to implement in your business since the therapist who learns more to bring to your practice will be motivated to earn more. If your income-earning power is less dependent on the therapist and more on what your business provides, and if the therapist has proven results with happy clients under your business name, you will have more success in retaining clients and therapists in your business. If you are giving your employee less than fifty percent of the money from services that are charged, you are not going to retain your therapists. It would be best if you strategize how to make more from each client rather than creating more sessions. This is the biggest change in mind-set that, if adhered to, will help make therapists happy and massage business owners more successful.

Empowering an employee and giving that employee the freedom to do what he or she does best is essential to your success. Properly qualifying those employees will be your best skill. And imagine if you could duplicate this model somewhere else? Making a profit in multiple places will give you the financial freedom you need to begin your process of retirement or allow you to work when you want to and not because you have to. MPB and Achieve Systems, which will be mentioned later has solutions to help you make this happen.

Your best success in expanding is with you and what you truly want in a business. If you don't know much about what that looks like, start with the basics.

- Write a diagram of your dream location and layout of your facility.

- Stipulate what types of services you will offer.

- Add in what you could offer to your clients beyond massage. What's important to you in your health and the health of your clients in your practice? Design a program that you can offer them that supports them.

- Review the common objectives and goals your clients are trying to achieve to determine your niche market.

- Look into functional medicine and aligning with practitioners who request and examine lab work so you can properly work with your client's medical professionals.

- Plan a space where you can hold community classes for your clients and your power partners' clients to get people to walk in the door and get to know your business while learning more about health and lifestyle management.

- Determine how much nutrition advice you can provide or offer without pushing products you can offer that help the client with inflammation, flexibility, and/or recovery. Create home kits or home care programs to sell and implement for accountability for the client and the massage therapist.

We offer a reference list of highly successful and complete programs that you can become educated about to offer your clients in our resources section. In the end, you have the power to create something great for your clients that doesn't take a large investment in terms of establishing yourself as a health professional. MPB provides over one hundred opportunities to help you build something great.

manifesting your future

WHEN YOU CREATE A BUSINESS in any industry, you create a business plan that essentially is the manifestation of your plans to make money. When we start out in the massage industry, we are focused only on how many people we can physically and emotionally see in a day; how many we "need" financially, offering packages that bring clients in; how to get clients; and how long it will take to get enough clients to pay for a professional space. While this thought process is OK, we need to change our thinking about that immediately since it will limit income potential. If you look around at all the storefront massage clinics and stores, you will see that many are capitalizing on how they can make money in our industry. The only difference between us building our business and them building a larger offering is they have a model in which everything is set up for earning money. Do you have a profitable business model like that? I didn't either.

It's simply because no one has ever attempted to show us how. However, you may happen to be a massage therapist with an entrepreneurial mind who has designed a practice that shows a profit and the ability to expand your location and duplicate this in another area. If this thought has never crossed your mind, you need to start thinking about the potential for it to come to fruition. What would it mean to you to earn enough money monthly to travel internationally, spend more time with your charitable causes, and still make money? It is possible. Unfortunately, business training is not mainstream in our industry. We are already set up to fail, according to recent statistics. According to an Earthlite blog in December 2015, an average of 50,000 new enrollments occur in massage schools every year, and 45,000 people leave the industry within the first three to five years due to burnout from working too hard to make money for someone else. The blog article, titled "5 Things to Consider When Going to School for Massage Therapy," indicates that injuries play a part in these statistics, too, since therapists are rarely trained in self-care. So they don't pace themselves in terms of the number of massages they can physically do in a day. Only five percent of graduates continue in the industry for the lifetime of their career.

The top reason people leave our industry is because of burnout and the inability to make enough money. Would you have burnout if you knew how to better structure your income? The answer is no. To have longevity in your career, you have to have the full picture to create the income you need and deserve. Doctors also have no idea how to have their practice run as a business. They hire managers to run their practices smoothly and to maintain the networks they need to funnel income into their offices. A doctor, who acts as a provider who bills insurance companies, has incentives and the network to see a large number of patients every day. We do not have this opportunity to hire people to manage our practices for us unless our model and business plan provides that for us.

Some therapists are sure that billing insurance companies is an excellent means to a higher income stream, which it can be. However, they are left to live in a box of attracting one kind of client—a client who relies on benefits through his or her insurance and not creating a strategy for better health. Those clients are not invested in long-term solutions. In such a case, it becomes challenging to provide for clients outside the high-dollar billing you have set for yourself in massage by billing through an insurance company. Be sure that is what you want to do to establish your income. Again, in our industry, we often need or want to change what we do, so be sure that when you get involved with insurance billing that you will enjoy it. I choose not to be part of the insurance model for various reasons, but mostly because people do not get well on their own if they rely on what an insurance company says they recommend to get better. I've chosen to work with clients who want to discover their wellness journey. They are looking for it, and they need it. Many massage therapists have to look to themselves to be a manager their practice because their income can't support hiring outside managers. If you bill insurance, you know how valuable it would be to have someone do your billing and management for you. Hiring a practice manager could become your reality if you would be open to examining what you need and want and implementing that for your business. Just be sure you will be able to make the income necessary to support this model and commit to it full-time. If you decide to bill insurance, your cash-client base will have to pay the rate you're billing insurance. It is illegal to bill insurance a different rate than your cash-pay clients.

How do you manifest your future? Create your business from the heart—for yourself, your clients, and the impact you want to make in the world. Create the income goals by manifesting what you need first and want second by writing it down. Your business plan will include these items and must reflect real goals. Make your financial goals emotionally motivated because as we work from the heart, we also have to create our goals with emotion. Otherwise, the goals have no meaning. A business plan has facts, but as massage therapists, we work with emotion every day, so we must create our plan with emotional outcomes. If you are charitable, list how your income can help your charity. If you are funding a college account for your kids or grandkids, list how your income can help fund those accounts and how great it would make you feel to have some income going toward a personally positive outcome. If you want to contribute more to your household because you want to do your part creating pride and support, establish what the income is, and incorporate it into your plan. What else motivates you to make income?

Creating more income is thinking outside the box. How can you provide more to your clients? It's time to leave behind your model of trading hours for income and instead create programs for your clients. Do not ever discount your rates, and do create additional income streams for yourself. What are additional income streams? Additional income streams are avenues of income that you incorporate to your career that have residual power to support you the rest of your life. These can be explored with Massage Practice Building, a company I created through Achieve Systems, the most comprehensive business support and coaching program available. You can learn more from visiting these websites, which are in our resource list. If you are anxious to begin creating your plan, start today by journaling your emotional motivators and incorporating them into your business plan. Have you noticed that you attract what you think about? You are powerful, and if your emotional thoughts are positive, they will bring positive out-comes. When you say, "I won't make enough doing massage," then you won't. If you believe what family and friends say about not making enough money, you won't. Maintain relationships that support your efforts, and dismiss others that work against you. If that person is your significant other, you will need to stay strong and state what it is that you need and how important it is for you to accomplish your goals.

Relationships often change as we get older because we constantly evolve through our lifetime. This is not a bad thing; it just leaves the traditional model of relationships a part of history. These are part of the past: when no one really talked about what help they needed, ignoring the ability and empowerment of creating their goals, not asking for and admitting to themselves what they needed, and never having the ability or the opportunity to accomplish more. As human beings in our current society, we sometimes can no longer maintain those traditions. If our significant other can grow with us, that is optimal. However, often when we discover who we truly are through doing this work, we do shed a part of us that no longer serves us. Sometimes they grow with us and sometimes they cannot. This may compromise some or all relationships we have. However, your evolution will ultimately take place, and it will change your priorities, just as it will change theirs. Journal about the situations, the relationships, and your thoughts in your everyday life and list both the positive and the negative. This is your self-assessment of your thought processes, and how they may be holding you back from your journey of success.

Incorporate positive thought into your business plan. It's essential for you to create and attract the community of help you need to be successful. Most of all, you may be able to create all of this on your own, but a community of support brings energy that will catapult you forward. This is true of any business, not just massage therapy. People need community to learn from one another, develop skills in business, and realize their full potential.

RESOURCES

- For strategic and comprehensive client development for massage therapists, we recommend the Massage Practice Building Workshop at www.massagepracticebuilding.com. Also, for advancement in the business of massage therapy—with resources to help every level of practice, including developing a clinic or wellness center—we recommend Achieve Systems at www.achievesystemspro.com/discover-achieve-catalogs.html.

- For customer relationship management (CRM) software, and for booking appointments, we recommend Genbook, which has a high-profile search engine optimization (SEO) result with Google. The more reviews you get, the higher up your listing becomes on Google. Others in the industry that are widely used for CRM are Full Slate and MassageBook. Research these and more that are available online. Some incorporate payment processing, newsletter features such as those offered by Constant Contact, prepayment options, online booking, appointment confirmations and reminders, charting, and push promotions. Decide which you will use for your client base and above all else do not pay too much. Most comprehensive programs run around forty dollars per month; if you spend more than that, review all the tools they provide and make sure you are using almost everything. If you are not, consider a provider that best suits your needs.

- For processing payments by credit cards, one recommended option is Square, the most user-friendly credit card processing company. However, once you start consistently bringing in $1,000 per month, look at other vendors who provide packages with varying rates. Others include Paystri and PayPal. Alternatively, you can check with your local small-business merchant processing companies. They are like brokers and can help you calculate your best method of processing based on your sales.

- A comprehensive coaching and business plan is essential to your success in today's massage therapy market if you want to make big things happen. It's here that you set your goals with your type of client, sales, location, pricing, sales forecasting, development, and future timeline for where it's headed. Continuing to strive for more without a goal is pointless. You need a written plan to support what you would like to manifest. Massage Practice Building (www.

massagepracticebuilding.com) and Achieve Systems (www.achievesystemspro.com) are your best resources to create your business for success. This will save you years of learning how to build a business for long-term success and additional income.

These are just a few resources to start with. There are many more, and plenty of support groups can help you. However, be careful about the money you spend on coaching from a business coach. These tend to be business oriented and have no experience in the massage industry. Expect support be given after the initial payment is made to coaching especially if you are paying five thousand to ten thousand dollars. Experts in our industry can tell you the best methods to use but only talk with those who are at a high level of income as these experts have learned to do it right in their own way. It may not be your way, but if they are a good coach, they will customize your learning process for your industry and give you full access to their tools and programs. Partnering with these people will be inspiring and give you the push to learn how to bring in a substantial income. A coaching system such as Achieve Systems is your best bet for meeting your immediate needs, future planning needs and accountability systems that keep you on track for a minimal monthly cost.

have
no
fear

THE ONE THING ABOUT BEING AFRAID in starting your business is that you are not alone. Everyone has fear when going out on his or her own, even in traditional business models. What is uncertain in our industry is that there are several recommendations and guides by various massage business leaders, but in the end, it's a matter of creating the best business model possible for returning the most life-sustaining income for you and your loved ones. You now have the business support you need to accomplish your success.

When business owners start out working for themselves, they have to gain an understanding of the processes of running their business. They write a business plan (to get a business loan from a bank), create their methods of running their business, and develop their goals for success within that plan. They describe what they offer, what they sell, hours of operation, location, marketing plans, market analysis, competition, and pricing. They set up the portrait of their business before they open their doors. Everything is planned and designed ahead of time. As skilled therapists, we also need to create this plan in owning our practice or business. What currently is happening is that massage schools turn out therapists without a plan whether they want to work for someone else or on their own. I have a mission to change this.

Some massage schools have good business training and might provide a short-term plan (not a long-term plan), but schools that don't give any instruction for their graduating students to work for themselves recommend working for someone else to gain experience. Well, guess what, folks? We are all equally capable of working at the same level right out of massage school. There is no reason to *have to* work for someone else since then your efforts reward someone else. If you are OK with that, be sure to keep your desire to work on your own in view, on a vision board or in your written goals. In our world, this is no longer the expectation of the first step in our career, though sometimes working for someone else does pay the bills. Be sure you set your goals right away with a plan to get out of working for someone else including setting a date to start full time on your own. You might also consider doing mobile massage and being employed at the same time so you can build your clientele. You must realize these goals in one to two years, or you will never make then change, or it will become increasingly more difficult to accomplish.

Why do we see so many therapists unhappy in the corporate massage chains environment? I'm sure you can agree that we could write several chapters on this issue. It only continues to happen because we all allow it. In many aspects of our lives, we need to be told a process of how to start out in our careers. Look back and see how this has occurred in your lifetime. When we finish school, we are not always empowered to strike out on our own unless we plan it, and in today's world of massage chains, *we can* stand out as businesses. Our schools need to enhance their curriculum to provide guidelines to success—not instruction that you "need" to work for someone else to get experience. These guidelines to success are hard to find in our industry right now. You can get experience without working for someone else; what you're missing is your confidence.

How do we gain confidence in any aspect in our lives? Experience! And in our case, that means hands-on experience. Have you ever been at a job interview where you are asked, "What's your experience?" And how many times do we say, "I'm here to get experience." We think that unless we work for free, we can't get experience, and we can't work for free because that doesn't pay the bills. So here you are discouraged and maybe feeling a little more vulnerable than you thought. So you find a place that will hire you, but that may not be in your best interests. From the start you may plan to leave, so how can you settle in anywhere if you already know you are going to be unhappy there? Dissatisfaction with doing sales for someone else is a common reason we got out of working for someone else and attend massage school. Making other people feel better is what we love, and selling is not. Someone might say, "I'll have to sell my skills to work for myself." Well, in a sense that is true.

But you are able to do that when you are happy doing what you love, when you lead with authenticity and when you have the skills with the service you offer. In our case, you have the training you need to do the work; what you are lacking is the permission and confidence you need to accomplish your plan. Your plan is *your* plan and never belongs to anyone else. Sometimes we go with what other people are doing. However, capturing what you want in your life and your business is yours to own.

And guess what? Every business owner has some fear around having success. This is when mentors become an important resource to tap into. We keep our fears in our cells when we don't own them. Yeah, I'm scared to get started. Yeah, I'm not sure I can help everyone. Yeah, I don't know if I'm good enough. Yeah, I don't know how I'm going to pay rent every month. These are all legitimate fears, so own them. And trust me; even those who appear confident starting out are not one hundred percent confident. However, because they present themselves as confident, people are drawn to them.

What it comes down to is this: Know that you have enough skills to start out on your own. People don't generally tell you that you *are* good at something if you really are not. If clients feel good and come back, you are good, and if they don't come back, then you need some mentoring from a successful massage therapist. Once you are licensed, you can earn money. Begin to practice on people and have a good plan to make money. Don't ever discount your services, even if you are new in the industry. It will take you years to make the income you deserve. The less you charge, the less you will attract clients to you since you are not displaying how valuable your work is. If you create the same routine for each client and never vary your offerings they will not get what they need and move on. Quite honestly you are doing them a disservice. It's your job to practice how to know what they need and implement ways to provide that for the client. Money is an energy exchange and means to survival so begin to embrace its value and yours in the process.

Here is a fact to consider in setting your pricing. In 1996 a one hour massage was placed at an average of sixty dollars per hour. Today you need to consider that sixty dollars in 1996 is the equivalent of ninety seven dollars and eighty cents in 2019. Think about how the cost of living has increased and yet the massage industry pricing for the private practitioner, in general, has not increased at all. Increasing the average rate in the industry is not about getting more money—it is about survival.

Get your plan together and jump! Jump in with both feet. Get that office space you like; your business plan will show it will work. There are lots of marketing strategies out there, but in the service industry, there is only one type of system that works—being good at what you do and showing confidence in yourself. With those skills and a massage health-care program for everyone, the fear will fall away, especially when developing your business for a specific type of client and not doing everything for everyone. Focusing on your niche will bring success in finding clients, and then helping others not in your niche will follow. The best strategy is to lead with your niche to get noticed. And in that niche, what makes you great? More training, more practice, and being creative and inventive. We are all artists, after all. Make something that people love.

Often we hear the statement, "It's easier to start working somewhere else. I can start my practice later." Delaying your desire to work on your own makes it harder to recapture the desire. The passion dies, and you will tend to settle in. When you are not on your own, you don't have the freedom to create your art as a massage therapist. Instead, you operate according to someone else's timeline and method of practice. Under those circumstances, you would not use what you know, control how you would spend time on your clients, and you might not provide the quality of care you can give them.

Do not delay your start. In our industry today, the perception of work opportunities in massage therapy is wrong. The industry perception favors the employer, the owner who entices you with offering benefits. In some cases, massage therapists just out of school need benefits, so it is seemingly essential for them to take a job as an employee. Break this mind-set now; it is possible to work what you need into your plan to pay your health care. If you have preexisting health conditions, this is a little more challenging, but there are plenty of resources out there. You just need help in finding them. In our industry, I hear graduates say their school told them to go out and get experience and then open their own practice once they have the experience. This is a *huge* problem with our industry. We are all equally qualified. Yes, you need experience, but you do *not* have to work for someone else and give your effort away for someone else's benefit.

Think about it. You are sacrificing your body's energy to put money in someone else's pocket, and you may develop pain and injury and lose time as a result of your efforts for someone else. You will need more bodywork (which you can trade if you know the right people), chiropractic help (mostly paid out of pocket), and rest (taking time) outside of work if you don't work at a pace that is comfortable for you. Before you consider applying anywhere, ask yourself, "How can I make enough money on my own to pay for my insurance, rent, expenses, and own compensation too?" Make a list of everything. No matter how much these things cost, don't worry about the dollar amount. Focus on how much you need to bring to your household. Take your mind-set away from "how can I" and focus instead on "this is how much I need to contribute." That will change what you are asking from the universe. It would help if you came from the land of plenty in your mind.

WHAT ARE THE NORMAL FEARS?

Am I good enough? Can I help this person? You won't know until you try. I am always nervous before every new client, even after twenty-three years practicing. This fear is a normal fear. Let it be OK to feel this way.

I feel if you maintain a certain sense of being humble, people will be drawn to you. At the same time, you must know your stuff. Find the balance of confidence and humility; it will reward you. In the end, your clients come to you and stay with you because you are part of their path to wellness delivered from the divine. Just like any relationship, it is meant to be. If they don't come back, someone else will fill their spot; it's that simple.

Become an expert in what you offer each client instead of counting how many clients you need. Coming from a place of need only maintains the underlying fear of what you doubt about your abilities as a business owner. Taking control of what you can in what you offer, how you offer it, and your skill set and knowledge behind it are going to change your mind-set. They will develop you as an expert in your own practice. People follow successful people, so create something with success that they can follow, and the people they know will also follow.

Your business will support you—*if* you have a plan. Businesses that don't have a plan fail. Businesses that don't have a realistic plan that is attainable will fail. If you are not sure if your action plans are realistic, reference our partner book: *The Ninety-Day*

Success Express Massage Therapists: A Proven System for Building a Client Base in 90 Days. There you will find answers to those questions.

I'M SCARED I CAN'T PAY RENT

Switch your focus. Your energy is going into the wrong place. Take control of that fear by creating more opportunities to make money. Have a chair massage gig at a client's office, or in any one month of the year hold a giveaway of gift certificates that have only three to six months to expiration (these have no monetary value and are tax deductible as a marketing expense). This gets people in the door and allows you to make an offer to someone new. There is a strategic plan we discuss in the Massage Practice Building Client Development workshop. Learn more at www.massagepracticebuilding.com. Make a plan to earn money without discounting.

As your business grows, your job description is CEO, owner, and provider. As you create your success, more of the management of your practice will be able to be outsourced. So let's get you to outsource your bookkeeping, accounting, client retention management, laundry, and whatever else that will help you have more time available to network, meet with people who bring your business and increase more offerings to your business.

Just as working for someone else is a stepping stone to a next job and any subsequent jobs in the future, starting your own business entails a need to take chances, make mistakes, and reinvent for a short period. Focusing on creating better health for your clients is the number one goal, and setting yourself up to succeed is equally as important. Over time, your efforts to create and maintain a system for your end goal—supporting you personally and professionally—is what makes your practice have its presence of success or failure.

matching your passion with reality

TRACK HOW YOUR PASSION TO SERVE matches with reality since what you already know helps you design programs for clients and helps you earn the money you deserve. The biggest downfall for massage therapists is in never increasing the value of what you do. You want to show yourself as an expert based on the results you get and the education you've gotten. Will you continue to take continuing education and yet not consider increasing your rates to reflect your expertise? Do you have a master's degree in massage? Are you a professor in massage? Recognizing the steps you have taken to advance yourself as a professional is essential to standing out in the industry. If your passion is to provide product with your treatment plan make sure you are seeking supplemental income that fits with your style of service. If it's a product that you manufacture and sell make sure you have the ability to exhaust your inventory, which your return on investment is high and you are making a profit. It may be that money becomes a constant quest and a constant distraction from creating something of your own to implement in your treatment. If you are asking yourself, "How can I make more money?" then look within and examining what you can offer other than an outside product. You are your best product! Your knowledge and your creativity are your best products. Selling outside product is OK only if it supports the treatment you provide.

Often I see therapists getting distracted by learning about MLM payout models when their focus on developing how a product or products aligns with their work and enhances the results their work brings to their clients. A product must be something you believe in not about how much money you can make in sales. In all aspects of your practice looking at where your passion and heart for enhancing a client's experience is vital for us; it's what drives us to love being massage therapists. If you don't love what you are doing, change it now! It will come through in your work and will reflect in the number of clients you are seeing. Why don't you love it? You need to explore why.

IDENTIFY YOUR PASSION

Throughout your career, you must look at your passion. What is your passion? In our profession, we usually say, "To help people feel better." While this is always true, what does that mean to you? What specifically can you do to make people feel better that is within the ethics and standards of our profession? Keeping in line with our passion will make us work naturally to earn more clients. Make this a journaling process if you need to. When we write our desires, they are concrete, and we can tie pieces together to stay in touch with ourselves. Dig deep. In your journal, answer these questions for yourself. Write out cases where you have made a large impact on a client if you want to see how you truly do help your clients. Even write one that was not as successful. This is a reality check.

- What is it you learned in massage school that gave you ideas about what you could offer your clients? If you are starting out, this is an easier question to answer than for those who have been in practice for a while. Looking at our first instincts is crucial to explore. Remember those thoughts and feelings that guided us in the desire to learn the art of massage therapy.

- Are these previous thoughts the same today? Look at the one class or technique you learned that really felt great to practice. Most likely what you thought you might have wanted to do has changed over time, and that's part of you building yourself as the artist you are. What makes our profession so amazing is that we can change and adapt what we do throughout our career. We are ever evolving in our work, and those elements we learn in various advanced trainings help us create the best melting pot of style we can imagine. Adding to what you provide to your clients is where you develop your best intuition. Creativity comes from intuition. You are using ten different techniques from four different trainings. That's great! It's at this point that we adapt to what the client needs and what makes us each unique. We often use these modalities or skills in all our sessions with all clients because it's organic and it flows easily through us. If you have learned something technical such as corrective techniques or stretching and these resonate with you, that is what flows through you and what the client needs since you have learned that skill and enjoy applying it to your work.

- What makes clients come back to you? Look at building more of these things if you are seeking more clients. What comments do your clients have that you can build on, that can build your confidence, and that can indicate what they love about you? Your success will grow from discovering what aspects of healing and what techniques you consistently apply that provide results.

- What happens when you finish a session with a client who sees results not once but multiple times? Find out what those results are, and be aware of what it is that makes you a great therapist for that client. If you don't know about the results, be sure to ask clients over time. Are their goals being reached? What are their goals? Many times clients become comfortable with you as a therapist, and that is great, but what is the next phase for their health journey? Come up with a question-naire for them to answer questions about how you help them. Just don't ask, "How am I helping you?" Design your questions around their growth. How do they feel physically, mentally, and spiritually? Are the relation-ships in their lives in a good place? Are they feeling more confident in their body, mind, and self-esteem? These are great questions for them to answer and understand in their health journey for themselves. You can gather this information to gain their trust and to use in the future in case their old patterns return.

- Why do clients come once and then never come back? A lot of times they are not look-ing at investing in themselves, or they don't have a health journey to lead. Depending on how much this happens, this might be painful, but it's so important for your reality check in knowing if you are really passionate about how you apply techniques and massage. In some cases, you may not have had the best training in school, which perhaps put you behind the curve. What can you do to improve that? Taking more classes in continuing education is the key to any successful career in massage therapy. You must know your anatomy, well! You must also know contraindications, very well! You must be able to read the clients well and know how to approach them and meet them where they are at. Looking at what you know and how you approach people is so important to your success.

- How finely tuned are your intuitive skills? Are you able to hear what the body is telling you, and does it match what the client is feeling? When you are working, and the body tells you something, are you engaging the client around it? Asking the client for feedback during a session when you get a feeling, a visual impression, or a question to ask is imperative to that client's healing journey. Clients can release old patterns by speaking about their past experiences or acknowledging what they are feeling in words. Could this skill be enhanced for you? Training in energy work and intuitive development will help enhance those skills. We have references on these modalities in our resource list.

- What is the reality for the client? Giving clients what they need and not what they expect are two different approaches. They can be the same, but as the practitioner, you can help them understand the difference. Some clients who see a therapist for massage and have seen someone else for years have an expectation. It's important for you to know what those expectations are and then see how they match with your style. If they are different, explain what it is about your work that brings results. The first session will be successful if you match their expectation yet give them your style with an effective treatment. They will immediately become more open to receiving your work. Hone in on what you do, write it down, and practice how you would explain it to new clients. Could they get a treatment from someone else the same way you deliver it? No, they couldn't. This is where your passion becomes a reality for the client. What they get from you they can't get from anyone else. Believe that, and make sure you are on the same page with the client. This confirms your passion for what you do and how you do it well.

You may explore these questions even if you are successful since it's always great to check in with how your passion meets reality. Self-improvement is why we are here.

IDENTIFY YOUR INCOME SOURCES

It's so much easier to look elsewhere for income. If you are not making enough money from bodywork, this is not a failure. It is not knowing how to make enough money in bodywork alone. Suppose you are thinking, "What am I doing wrong?" That is not the question to ask yourself—*ever*! Believing that you are doing something wrong is negative and not good for your spirit. Instead, focus on things you are doing right. Seeking additional income is great for the long-term, but first, you must capitalize on what you can offer that is helpful and positive in helping your client. If you have experience in other forms of preventive care, focus on this and have the proper information to share with your client. Be sure to ask if your clients are open to learning something about it before you tell them. Otherwise, they won't be listening. If you don't have links to such information or have libraries of research to refer to, have some book recommendations for them or have a lending library in your office. This is an example of using what you know to help your client.

If you are seeking income outside of you such as through MLM companies that sell essential oils, nutritional products, home care products, or all of these, stop and reevaluate your thought process. Ask yourself if the time you need to spend learning about a product will yield the result you want when you have a client on your table. Many of them sound like a great source of additional income but tread lightly. Make sure that taking more time to sell products than you spend with clients is something you want to do. Some of it sounds too much like sales, so make sure you keep this in mind as clients come to you to feel better and will do what you recommend in the form of bodywork. Yes, nutrition is critical, and nutritional products will align nicely with your practice. However, know your facts and be sure you can give them information about nutrition and not act as a nutritionist. In some states that is not within your legal scope of practice. So why not participate in MLM? There are some great products out there, but the priority for a therapist revolves around skill and creativity in the massage offered and in the tools to make additional income related to massage therapy. This is the reality. Selling products as additional income will take you only so far, and clients get burned out on products, especially if they don't help them like we hoped they would. I know some therapists do really well with selling products. Why? Because they believe in it so much that it becomes their passion, and that is great! But selling products doesn't work that way for all massage therapists because it's not their passion, and the client's lack of interest will deflate the excitement. What lands a client is the skills you have in your hands that provide the client results. Develop yourself as a practitioner, but not in product sales. There are great MLM products out there, and I don't discourage therapists from selling them. However, they are a distraction in most cases because the person who signs you in is most interested in your sales performance because that person gets paid on your efforts and will constantly check in to know if you need help selling products. If you can provide the products and sell them organically, that is the best approach. Otherwise, focus on how to make money within what you know and provide as a massage therapist. What do you already tell them to do in between appointments that could be considered coaching?

What generates the flow you need in your practice to attract clients is the same as what successful representatives in MLMs are great at—establishing relationships. So you will need to ask yourself, "Where will I make the most money in establishing relationships?" If it's not in your practice and your passion for helping others with your work, you definitely need a reality check on how you are offering your services. You are not matching your passion with reality because your focus has turned to a product-based practice. We have the opportunity now more than ever to create programs for our clients. Think about what that could look like for you, and capitalize on the end goal of helping clients through their health journeys and goals. This will make you a respected and unique therapist.

CREATE YOUR INCOME

How can you set your pricing to your full potential? We are in a market where we must differentiate ourselves from the average massage experience and pricing reflects how we attract business. We have witnessed where CEO's and high-income earners will never seek a seventy-dollar massage. They look for a high priced value. This does not mean you cannot price something to meet lower income earners; you must have something for everyone. Mostly we are not in this business for the money because we love what we do, and we don't often think about our needs for income first. By doing this, we are matching our client's expectations of an affordable massage—not thinking of our own survival. Did you know as a massage therapist you don't need a second household income or second job to sustain your lifestyle? There are CEOs all over the world who pay themselves extremely well because they define their own income. Why don't you? If you are, then that is awesome! We often base our rates on what others charge. The biggest controversy and disharmony in our industry is what others are charging for massage. Don't get caught up in what others charge. Do what *you* need to do to establish your own value based on the income you need to support yourself and your family. Be your own professional. If you choose to stay on the low end for people to see you, then that's OK. However, know that you will continue to struggle to make ends meet while you have the market and the ability to create more income for your future. It is a choice. To establish your rates, you have several aspects to consider:

- How good are you at what you do? Do you provide results every time? How do you know what these are? If you rebook every client consistently over long periods of time, you are an amazing provider who provides your clients results.

- How many hours of base training from massage school did you have, and are you satisfied with the education you received? If you did not spend extra time on anatomy, physiology, and kinesiology and its application to the body, this must be a priority, especially when working with medical professionals. Hone your knowledge and skills to create more value for a better result.

- What have you taken in continuing education that can create more value for you? Taking a variety of courses allows your skills to improve and enables you to create your own style, not to mention that those courses help make you a masterful massage therapist.

- What percentage of your income goes to rent? Rent can be painful, but it's necessary for those who don't have a house in which to set up their business. Often office spaces are more convenient to the majority of your clients. Raising your rates because of increasing costs is not unreasonable. Do your clients get raises at their jobs? Why can't you?

- Do you spend a lot of time with your client instructing that client on lifestyle changes, stretches, home exercises, and a helpful ear? This is a value that we do not learn in terms of how to apply it to our services. You don't need to nickel-and-dime per minute or hour. Just present it in your pricing as a value of your time.

- How many clients can you see in a week? Sixteen to twenty is full- time for some while twelve to fifteen is full-time for others. Regardless of the number of hours you can work on bodies, design your income based on hands-on work first, instruction and coaching second, and outside product sold third. Your end income will be what is made per client and not what is made per hour. Focus on what you can earn per client.

- What do you need to bring home after expenses and taxes? This is key in factoring what you need to make to live comfortably and have the ability to save for retirement, have vacations, and take continuing education classes. Don't forget what you need to save for paying quarterly taxes.

Regardless of what you think you should charge, your base minimum starting rate should be determined by where you live. In Los Angeles, Chicago, and New York, of course, rates are high because of their high cost of living. If the cost of living and trends in the marketplace in your area have increased dramatically in the last few years, you need to increase your rates along with these trends. You often see this in the prices of housing. As these increase, so will your rates. None of us likes price increases on anything, but this is reality. The value of the dollar in 1996 has declined to the extent that a one-hour massage that cost sixty dollars then would cost $97.80 in today's dollars. Clients will understand your rate increase, but if they don't, ask them about the last time they got a raise. And how many raises have they had in the last three to five years? It's simple. They must know this is your full-time job, and you don't do it just because it's fun. You are allowed to set the tone in establishing your rates. If you increase your rates, don't continually increase five dollars at a time. Increase in fifteen-dollar to twenty-dollar increments. If they can't afford that, then grandfather them in for a period of time. We struggle with this because the people who really need the help are out of work for physical reasons and have little income for their care. In that case, put them on a payment plan to see you. A great coach and mentor I have says, "Always make a program for everyone." You know your own path, and if you are OK with making the minimum for your entire career, that is your choice, of course.

This advice is for those who struggle with not making enough to survive independently and continue to avoid raising rates for years. These are tips for massage therapists who need to develop themselves as business owners and future clinic owners.

you're a professional

ESTABLISHING YOURSELF AS AN EXPERT in advising your clients is essential to your professionalism and credibility as a practice/business owner. These relationships are available to everyone. A successful therapist is one who recognizes a client's lifestyle and how it impacts that person's physical and emotional being. Notice how your various clients have imbalances in mind, body, and/or spirit. Look at what client you tend to draw in. Do you have what it takes to take care of clients who have a lot of drama in their lives, or do you attract clients that need physical help or both? What percentages need emotional support versus physical support? It's important to understand this since you need to recognize your strengths in what you provide. We all can help everyone, but this process of recognizing what organically suits you is essential for your development as a therapist and the development of your business. As a quality practitioner, not only do your skills need to be top-notch but your knowledge of what impacts the client emotionally and physically needs to play a part in that client's total wellness and give him or her the best tools to use in daily life. This can substantially vary based on the client. We tend to attract clients who are encountering similar emotional and physical challenges to those we have faced. Based on their intuition about our own experiences, they subconsciously seek us out to help them because we understand what they are feeling. Stay within your scope of practice when giving advice by stating your experience. But don't divulge too much personal information, and use only reliable resources for your small touches of advice. I suggest start by saying, "Are you open to hearing something about what I think might be going on with you?"

Alternatively, you might say, "When I went through this…" or "In my experience…" If you don't know exactly what the client may be experiencing, say that you will do some research. Have a few counselors lined up whom you can refer to if need be. Here you show concern, and you learn more information for yourself along the way.

PHYSICAL

Knowing the body's systems and its functions has to play a part in your client's care. You don't need to know everything, but you need to know enough to have a conversation with the client based on the client's lifestyle. Use the information you learned in school about the science of the body and how the body uses kinetic and cellular energy. Know your anatomy and how movement and injury affect the body. If you didn't have enough training, seek out more training through continuing education, massage therapy books, and anatomy reference books. Use verified online resources for a quick reference when needed. Also look at your clients' spiritual paths and how their struggles in life are related to their current state of mind and body. Clearly, they are searching for solutions if they are coming to see you. If you don't know these things right now, that's OK. Read up on somatics, or better yet, use your professional power partners and experienced massage therapists as a resource for information.

EMOTIONAL

You cannot, within your scope of practice, diagnose or act as a counselor to your client unless you have a license to practice counseling. You can be a good listener and help the client based only on your own positive outcomes in the form of your emotions related to healing your body, but nothing more than that. The most important thing is a good referral system to provide your client with the best counselors and therapists in your area. Checking in with your clients is needed from time-to-time, but know your professional boundaries, so that you are caring as a professional and not as a friend. When clients are vulnerable, you don't want to appear available outside your practice or office except to provide referrals. The clients' most vulnerable positions are on the table. If they are open to processing their emotions while they are receiving body-work, make sure you are prepared to listen and let them create their own process. To give them any advice at that moment takes away their self-discovery. You must be cautious in this situation. When a client is on the table, you as a bodyworker are in a position of great influence and power. (Even if you think you aren't, you are.) A client is very vulnerable here. Be aware and cautious, and he or she will respect you more if you stay neutral during moments when they are releasing through verbalizing, crying, or expressing anger.

I often hear from new clients that the therapist they saw previously had spilled out all their personal information, drama, and frustration on their client. This must not happen. Ever! It is so important to present yourself as a professional by limiting what people know about your life and your personal information. If you share too much about yourself, you will lose your credibility. If you are tenderhearted and don't stay neutral during their emotional release, it will hinder their process.

On the other hand, if you are too abrupt and matter-of-fact, you might seem uncaring, so you might need to tap into a softer side to show you care and make a connection. Taking ethics courses is essential to staying on task in keeping healthy boundaries with clients. Having your own emotions in check is even more important to providing quality work and being fully present for the client.

Keeping our troubles to ourselves is essential, and we need to promise to do this to protect our clients. It is one thing when a client asks you about how you are doing while on the table. It's OK to respond, keeping it brief and without drama. That's vital, and it keeps the boundaries clear, creating client respect for you as a therapist and not as a friend.

SPIRITUAL JOURNEY

Not only are you experiencing your complete spiritual journey outside your practice, but you are also learning that journey through your clients and their experiences. In our line of work, we understand how we are here to help others. It is a calling from the divine—no matter what your religious belief. A sense of knowing is what we draw on at all times. It's a skill we are born with and develop as practitioners. I graduated from the Boulder School of Massage Therapy in 1995. I came from a corporate environment where I was very cut off from connecting with people spiritually—except with what faith I grew up with. I had never meditated before or had any spiritual experiences until

I learned from my classmates at that school. I had classmates who had all kinds of spiritual gifts, and one classmate, in particular, told me how I had healing light all around me. I didn't feel it or understand it. I believed her, but I honestly had no idea what she was talking about. Other classmates had feelings of physical release and healing taking place when we worked on one another. It took a couple of years of practicing massage to recognize these experiences. I continued to learn about the spiritual energy connection the longer I had my hands on someone. Our spiritual journey is learned with those we touch; developing the skills is vital to your longevity and desire to do the work. I almost quit practicing during three life-changing events, and each time I talked to myself about changing my career, I knew I had to figure it out somehow. The work became my journey, and I knew as hard as it was to survive financially and professionally, my journey was tied to the work, and I couldn't quit. I also knew that the number of people who needed my help was increasing, and to watch them transform as they took their spiritual journeys while we worked together was a beautiful and rewarding experience.

Watching them discover more about themselves is only something we facilitate. We don't ever need to force their experience; it happens naturally. You may have already attained the skill and know it, or you may not know you have the skill. The only way you know is if clients are dedicated to seeing only you for massage. Enhancing your touch naturally happens once you practice for a number of years and open up to learning healing modalities and skills. It isn't mandatory, of course, to explore these, but you will begin to learn more about your purpose by exploring what you are here to do. Homing in on your intuitive skills is part of being successful. Exploring these modalities will root you in your work, and people will be amazed at how great you are. The divine provides clients as well, so if losing a client ever disappoints you, know there will be another to take that client's place. You still need to know how to draw clients but exploring yourself, your journey, and how you help others will help design how they come to you. Remember, though, you can't just sit and wait for them to show up; that isn't the reality. Your skills in your journey are essential, but equally essential is your ability to be smart about how to attract clients to your business.

CONTINUING EDUCATION

Our fifty states are constantly changing the massage laws concerning requiring continuing education to maintain a license, but don't let that stop you from learning. If you have graduated from massage school and no longer learn more to improve your skills implies that you are no longer interested in learning for your clients and/or learning to enhance your value. Do not seek continuing education solely online. While in school, didn't we learn best while working on one another and with one another? Your learning process will be much richer if you enroll in classes. As the profession has gone online with education, we have been losing touch with one another, literally and figuratively, of course. In general, we have disconnected from one another as professionals unless we have attended conventions or have been active in groups on social media. Online learning helps us as introverts. However, it takes away from developing our networking skills, a highly effective skill in enhancing our success in business.

What I have seen more of are therapists who don't want to invest in themselves, especially in states that don't require continuing education credits to maintain their license. I know it isn't easy. As I branched out into the role of serving as a leader to improve our industry, I had to battle my introverted nature. My passion for helping all therapists have equal opportunity has been a driving force in casting away my introverted side and expressing my extroverted side. I spent a lot of time learning what is needed in our industry, and I did that through networking with other therapists and health professionals and using my professional experience of twenty-three years as a reference. As hard as it can be financially for some of us, enrolling in classes is essential to our growth and development as professionals. It's easier not to, but how does that serve our clients' experiences and our experiences in life? Think about ways you can start networking with therapists, professionals, and yes, even business people. Every contact you make is for a reason. Staying back and waiting will not serve you or your clients. We need to receive learning more to open up the possibilities.

ANATOMY AND KINESIOLOGY

Knowing anatomy and kinesiology is one of the most crucial components of being a therapist who is respected by other professionals. If you don't know your basic anatomy and muscle function, you are at a huge disadvantage in helping your clients properly and being able to appropriately discuss with other power partners your client's condition. For the more science-minded therapists, it is natural to know anatomy well. For those who barely passed anatomy and physiology in massage school and on the national exam, knowing all the muscles and bones may have become a less important part of participating in client care. That's because anyone's routine can become set in stone, with no variation, if the massage therapist allows it. If you lack the ability to name all muscles in the body, don't worry. You are not alone. If you can't name the major muscle groups and the key movers, then get out those old books, find new ones, look online, and download apps to find them. Find a client or another therapist who will take the time for you to palpate and know the muscle groups and their basic functions in everyday movement. Better yet, take a technical, hands-on class. Even with quality education under your belt, you might have difficulty remembering everything after massage school. If you are in sports and medical massage, you can't provide the right treatment without that knowledge, and you can't talk to doctors, surgeons, chiropractors, physical therapists, and trainers properly. The same goes for oncology care. You can't properly serve the client without knowledge of the invasive nature of breast cancer with respect to muscles, movement, and the lymphatic system, especially in the case of a mastectomy. Without that knowledge, you won't be serving the client at all. These are the basic principles of showing yourself as an ethical practitioner. Taking time and money investing in advanced education will elevate your presence and your confidence.

Part of a new movement in our industry is learning about functional medicine and functional testing. This is a service to the client you provide through your understanding of how the body functions. That enables you to direct the client to the right doctor or another practitioner, and it gives you the language you need to know how to speak with physicians. This is a huge step forward in our industry regarding presenting ourselves as professionals. Networking with and learning from these professionals will only give you higher value with your clients. Find resources to help you do this. We have included many in the resource pages that we will share with you.

personal presentation

IN OUR WORLD, WE TEND ALWAYS to be free-spirited and expressive, and it is in those modes that we are truly authentic. We often express our free spirit in what we wear, how we act, and what we have in our surroundings. As noted previously, I went to massage school in Boulder, Colorado. Boulder is known as a hippie town, and it's pretty cool, really. I didn't live in Boulder, but it has a vibe that is quite attractive to the inner hippie. There are many other towns like this across America, and we love that, don't we?

Some of us are drawn to the hippie lifestyle, dress, and culture since it offers a safe place where people accept one another for who they are and have no judgment about what others do. This makes sense since we cannot be judgmental of the clients we work with. I traveled to Boulder nearly every day for a year—a sixty-eight-mile round trip experience for forty weeks. I was disappointed to go back to a more conservative culture after my Boulder immersion since that was my safe place, where people accepted me as I was. Going back to "judgment town" felt like I had to look "right" to attract clients in downtown Denver—still a very casual place but not happy about hippies in 1995. That acceptance came many years later when the marijuana laws passed and gave Denver a relaxed mind-set.

My perceptions about the look of professionalism were a little skewed as I learned what others thought. Clients weren't highly concerned about attire, but you did need to look and smell clean. The most important things in professionalism are not what you wear or how you look, but you do need to meet your client's expectations. You need to create yourself, your office, and your space to be in sync with your goals as a practitioner and the type of client you want to attract to your business. This means planning from the inside out. In our industry, I'm noticing a lot of questions around what we should wear, and it seems therapists just need some permission for some to do what they inherently know and others to confirm that their choices were good ones.

If you are trying to attract CEO clients, have the proper attire to attract them. Your office appears sleek, updated, and clean. In other words, have a business-professional-looking setting. If you are trying to attract athletes and medical massage clients, your setting would include room for more equipment, such as foam rollers, bands, and floor mats for analysis of movement and workouts and anatomy posters you can reference. If you are part time and don't have a niche base of clients, then you have a little more freedom in creating your surroundings. The tone of your office may be more expressive, with things that enhance your work but still have an aura of professionalism. So you can even have your tapestry, prayer flags, and whatever enhances the healing process for you and your clients and appear professional.

TIPS AND SUGGESTIONS

- In all cases, if you are tuning into energy for your work, surround your office with those things that bring you that energetic connection. Tools that clear energy from the room—such as bells, chimes, bowls, incense, and sprays—are important to some but not everyone in clearing energy between clients. These are tools that clients might be interested in learning about. If you don't use energy clearing regularly, I highly recommend it. It is a form of self-care. Protecting yourself from lingering energies from others is important to our well-being and preventing burnout.

- Have sufficient space in your office for a reception area. Professionalism in any profession has an area of reception where you wait for your appointment, a place where the client is welcomed when the practitioner and the room are ready. This shows boundaries as well. You are not available on the client's time, but you always start on time. An example would be an instance in which a client becomes so comfortable with you that he or she passes straight through the reception area and walks right into your treatment room. A good practice is to close the door until you are ready. Make sure the clients know you will be with them shortly and that they can wait in the reception area. Even if you don't mind when they barge in, it's a great practice to hold them at a distance, and it creates their respect for your professionalism. Too many times upon entry, their energy is rushed or invasive, so this method is a way to get a client to collect, breathe, and arrive before he or she gets on the table. You are helping both of you by allowing the chaotic energy to dissipate before the session begins.

- If a client is late and your appointments are not booked too close together, you can choose to make an exception, but know that if you do this you will become a doormat to your client and create a bad habit of the client arriving late. Make sure to stick to your timeline on your calendar, so your clients know your time is valuable. In addition, do not discount your service—since you booked the full rate at the full time—even if it's a gift certificate. If the client is new, this is especially important to uphold since he or she needs to know you are a professional. You set the tone. If the client doesn't like your policy, don't worry. You will find someone else, and there are plenty of clients out there for you if you are good at what you provide. Let's put this into perspective. You wouldn't see a doctor going over the allotted time with a patient, so why would you? Moreover, you wouldn't stop seeing that doctor immediately either; you would wait because you would know that it would be hard to get back in for another appointment. If you do go over your time, as this often happens, it is OK to have conversations with your clients while they are on the table about going over another fifteen minutes but needing to charge them another fifteen dollars (or whatever is in line with your rate structure per minute). Your clients must respect your time, and you must equally respect theirs. If you are running late on appointments, text your clients and ask their permission to start the appointment fifteen minutes late if they have the time. Nothing is more annoying than waiting without having any information. Doctors' offices do this all the time, and I'm sure you can agree that not knowing a timeline in a waiting room is un-nerving. When you start an appointment late, always ask your clients if they are pressed for time; it shows respect for them, which helps them develop respect for you.

- Clients like us for how we dress as long as we don't wear anything too revealing or smell of perfume, cologne, smelly clothes, excessive essential oils, or body odor. Excluding those exceptions, they typically have no judgment. If you don't have a great sense of smell, you need to ask someone if you're giving off odors. If a smell is strong and makes clients uneasy, they will not relax during treatment, will never tell you, and may not return to see you.

- If you are really great at what you do, what you wear is not of great concern. There is much debate in the industry about presentation and what one should wear while working. First and foremost, always be comfortable, but it's equally important to be professionally dressed. This means different things for different areas of the country. New York and Chicago expect much more in their daily dress styles, maintaining an expectation that the massage therapist be fully and professionally dressed. Colorado and California, on the other hand, are much more casual—Colorado with jeans and California with shorts. Shorts are OK as long as they aren't cutoffs. If you live in an environment that is humid and hot, of course, you are going to want to wear something light, and if you are in a cold environment, you are going to often dress in layers. If we go to polo shirts and khakis, which is standard in clinical environments, we might feel too conforming and not true to our spirit. Men, you may not care so much about this, and polo tops and jeans or khakis may be standard for you. And may I say that you are blessed not to have to think twice.

- So find your comfort style. Graphic tees are fun if they have positive messages or represent you and what you love. Skirts are OK if they are long; tank tops are OK as long as your bra and your breasts are not making their own greeting. Camisoles are not recommended; we need to be conscious of what we portray. And ladies, if you are busty, cover up. We are at a point in American culture where anything goes, and the workplace is not the place for revealing too much skin, especially in our industry. I'm saying this because of what I've seen over the last twenty years, and what I know about problems occurring because of too much showing. It's best to be a bit more conservative.

- To the men, I'm sorry public perception of our industry has not reached the point of accepting you as equal providers in massage therapy. This is one of the most upsetting factors for all of us since there are so many *great* male therapists. It is essential, however, that you too have the appearance of professionalism. Hopefully, soon the perception will change, but it's an uphill battle with all the bad seeds out there. There are women offenders, too, but we don't hear about them as much. Unfortunately, when clients are selecting male or female therapists in spas or chain stores, most will pick females. Overall, to play it safe, you are smart to work for yourself in a professional office and have the ability to show your professionalism on your own. Connect with successful male therapists in the industry to help guide you throughout your career. Plenty are successful, so learn how they did it so you can continue your passion with success.

- Create your space to have comfort. Always have water available. Blankets are a very comforting offering since some clients like the weight of one or maybe need some extra warmth. Have a blanket that's heavy or medium weight and also one that's lighter for those who don't need that much warmth. I've been in plenty of massages where the air conditioning was very high because the therapist was too hot, but yet the therapist didn't have a blanket to offer. Have a table warmer under your table cover, so it remains sanitary. Offer it for everyone, and you will get to know which clients like heat and which do not. Some states have sanitary laws, so first make sure you comply with those laws. Have different-sized pillows for side work—a fluffy one for the head to fill shoulder space and a thinner one for a little bit extra bolstering, a neck roll or a towel, and body pillow. I use a body pillow I created. It is two body pillows stuffed into one body pillowcase. Body pillows today are not made for much support. Your pillow needs to be big enough to bring the femur parallel to the table. If it's not parallel, the pillow isn't big enough. Place another pillow to accomplish this. For busty women who need support when face down, roll a regular towel to place under their bra line for support. Use two hand towels folded under shoulders while the client is facedown to raise shoulders up so that you get better access to rhomboids and infraspinati. Use a rolled-up towel under the neck for support when faceup. These are a few comforts that you may already know clients love.

- Implement noise control. One of the hardest components in finding an office setting for clients is noise control. Noise happens, but you can do your best to make your space as soundproof as possible. Don't be afraid to ask for modifications. This is something negotiable with a landlord. We had white-noise vents installed in our office, which is the best solution for anyone. If your landlord is unwilling to do this for you, it's either time to find one that does, or you can bring in a stand-alone white-noise machine to buffer noise in your building.

There is a complete protocol in looking for space, reviewing leases, and knowing what questions to ask. In most cases, if the landlord isn't willing to adapt your space to your needs, then the landlord isn't open to having you there. It is common for landlords to want certain types of tenants instead of blending different industries in their buildings. While staying within budget is helpful, just know that you get what you pay for in the building you are in. Be cautious always, know the terms inside and out on your lease, and ask questions before signing. Your rent will go up every year. If it doesn't, you're lucky!

- If you are leasing space in a public building, you will likely have solicitors who enter your suite. If you don't have a receptionist, keeping the exterior suite door to your office locked is highly advisable to keep building foot traffic at a minimum, and it's also a safety measure for you and your client. It is always surprising when someone enters a suite and yells, "Hello," when the doors have signs that say, "Massage in Progress" or "Quiet Please." I'm sure some of you have experienced this. We have a policy to lock our door when we are in session unless we are booked tight, in which case we place a sticky note on the door that states, "Please leave door unlocked. Thank you." Creating a peaceful space is also providing a place of healing. Also, remember to tell your clients that sometimes the door will be locked and that they can wait in the lobby or work out an arrangement of texting to notify you that they have arrived. Included rules for this quiet space should be that cell phones need to be silent and vibration alerts need to be turned off. A good solution for this is to have clients put phones in airplane mode. Even vibration alerts disrupt the true relaxed state of the brain. The human brain has an automated response even when we sleep that reacts to any noise or energy coming from a cell phone. For personal use, keeping cell phones out of your bedroom is a good practice not only to keep the brain at rest but also to keep electromagnetic magnetic fields, or EMFs, away from your body as much as possible. Provide this precaution to your clients in your sessions as well.

- Your music selection should be in line with what your client wants—not what you want. I have several who don't like native drums, one who likes silence, and one a fountain. Always adapt to your client's comfort when you first come into the room to start the session. Asking if your clients are comfortable is an easy question and will give them permission to ask for something they need. They won't ask unless they are good about asking for what they need. You are the facilitator, not the person in power, in each of your sessions. You will find a client will have more open experiences and a better quality of healing if you always make the session about the client. Good communication and remembering what makes the client comfortable is the key to success in client retention.

- Be aware of where your body is in relation to your client. If you need to get closer to your client to accomplish treatment when he or she is clothed, let the client know as you go that you need to get close. While under a sheet, the client has little control over feeling safe from being exposed. In school, we undressed nearly every day for one or two years, and we tended to learn to be less modest. We've been covered only by a sheet so many times that I think we forget to be more conscious of a typical client's modesty. It is often overlooked in everyday practices. I've often been in a session with a therapist who brushed body parts up against me and leaned on me without notice, and all I kept thinking was this: What if I didn't know anything about how massage therapists love touch and tend to be less spatially aware? So be sure you have clear space between you and your clients until you get to know them better and *always* use two hands during your massages. Announcing that your techniques include your body touching them is a great piece of communication. You will almost never have anyone who is not OK with it unless the client is uncomfortable being on the table or is modest. If modest, make sure your draping techniques are top-notch. And if some clients are really modest, allow them to leave their clothes on. There are several training techniques that are effective with a client who remains clothed.

You may have your own methods you use that create comfort, and you may have an office setup that is agreeable for your client. Keep using what works, but consider some of these ideas if they apply to you and your clients. As I mentioned, some therapists are not sure what is allowed. A lot of what we learn is from one another. Working in a shared office space is a benefit in terms of learning and adapting your offerings accordingly. More importantly, what you find comforting in a massage or what you have seen in a colleague's office space that you love can be brought in any time for your clients. Creating that safe, secure place for healing and results is the ultimate goal. If you are creating the image of yourself as an expert and an excellent therapist, having the appropriate space for your clients will keep them coming back. But don't ever forget who you are, and if you tell your clients who you are, they will enjoy that part of you. We never want to come across as perfect; we only will have success if we are authentic.

healing
in the body

UNDERSTANDING YOUR MOTIVATION in helping others heal is essential to your success. Why did you apply to massage school? Most of us loved receiving a massage and wanted to help others feel the effects of massage and its great health benefits in the prevention of disease and illness. Some of us come out of school totally jazzed and ready to start while some of us need a vacation. We know how overwhelming a comprehensive program can be. We know how it can test our maximum tolerance for dealing with emotional issues and the mind-taxing content from anatomy and physiology that we cram into our brains in a short amount of time. As we come out of school, we work fervently with the body as we continue to learn how we can apply the different modalities that we learned. The more we practice with different body types, the more we learn how we adapt to what they need and being constantly grateful and surprised at what we encounter in each massage session.

With gratefulness comes growth in yourself and openness to receiving more clients whom you will help. As you develop your niche and master your craft over the years as an independent practitioner, you will have the ability and the time to devote to understanding how long it takes for the body to process the work you do. Learning how to keep seeing a client and learning how to refer out a client will bring respect to you as a professional because, in the end, it's about what the client needs. Until you work with other professionals with different modalities, you won't truly be able to see how integrative other modalities are for your clients. Those other modalities can help their end goal of healing and can give them a better quality of life. They might include Feldenkrais, prenatal, sports, medical, qigong, craniosacral, Reiki, Healing Touch, meditation, and almost anything that interests you with respect to learning more about the body.

GIVING TO THE CLIENT

Giving a client what he or she needs is missing in our industry today. Having higher skill levels, knowing the importance of nutrition and hydration, and using functional medicine as part of your care is what the client needs. Remember, you are the expert, and you know what clients need or the possibility of what they need. Your intake of each client will help you satisfy that need versus want as you work with the client over time. Pushing clients to their limit is not the approach, but setting a goal for them and getting to reach a little further is what you strive for in getting them well. This will come as you get more experience as a therapist, and you will notice you will draw in those clients for whom you adapt your treatments to meet their end goal.

We also know the results of trauma to the body for a client physically, emotionally, and sometimes spiritually. We call that "issues in the tissues." Clients may lose faith in themselves and a higher power that leaves them with questions of "why me, why now, and how am I going to get through this?" Moreover the body is what holds those beliefs. It's up to us to connect these issues with the tissues, empower the clients again, give them confidence, and have the time with them to support them in the moment. Time for the body to process what it receives is on the body's time and not ours. If we are watching the clock in order to try to get everything in that needs attention, time may be our nemesis. Going over on time can be bad for your business if you only book sessions fifteen minutes apart, and not going over on sessions can be a disservice to the body's process and healing. As you work with your clients individually and get to know them, their lifestyles, and how their bodies respond, you will know more about the pace you need to set in each treatment. Buffer your time between clients to the best of your ability. Allow this to be part of who you are as a therapist and part of your style of bodywork. You will continually be refining how the information you receive from the client and their body guides you through its process.

I've had plenty of times where I was certain I knew how a new client would respond to treatment, but as soon as I was certain, I was proven not in control every time because I was not in control; the body was. Being accomplished in this part of your business comes with time. Refining your time skills inside and outside your practice is your process of learning your business and the limits on your maximum offering.

HOW DO I KNOW HOW TO ORGANIZE MY DAILY SCHEDULE?

While it's important to keep your day running on time, you can be generous with your time between clients. Usually, thirty minutes between sessions is best. In our chapter "Personal Presentation," our suggestions on time become blurry when you have to allow the body to process new information that you are providing it. Using your best judgment and communicating appropriately with clients will always be well received. Taking care of you in the process is wise as well. Have plenty of snacks and nourishment on hand, and if you need time to gather yourself, allow your next client to get on the table and give that client the time to settle in and relax (unless the client needs to leave right at the end of the time scheduled). It's good to give yourself a meditative moment, a snack, water, or whatever else you need. If you make this a good practice, you will prevent burnout in the long run. As you create this environment, your practice will hold higher value. Therefore, create programs with higher value. In the end, though, aren't you providing what *they* need to have a higher-value experience? Won't you be a more respected practitioner, and won't you be well sought out for providing that for them?

This is the point that divides the line between a professional and a caregiver who is also a professional but may not offer as much value. The caregiver practitioner will be the person who has positive impact on a client by being a great sounding board, a facilitator of relaxation, and someone the client can count on to keep happy. The client comes in for the same condition every appointment, and that's OK, too, as it could be for chronic conditions that never have the possibility of improvement. But never limit yourself to that thought; the best nutrition and hydration can help them tremendously too.

At one point, the massage might give them the neurological retreat the brain needs, but is that enough? If you are seeing clients over and over for the same condition, and the massage is not helping, offer more or refer them to your other health partners, who are willing to work with your clients. Their progression is your mutual end goal.

PROVIDING MORE

Should we also be able to provide more to everyone in the form of life coaching, nutrition, and meditation? And should we help them develop a routine in which they can be accountable? Many people need constant quality care in the form of comfort, but in the end they need more of your expertise in what you know about the body's ability to heal better with quality nutrition, regular and plentiful water consumption, healthy surroundings, daily practices, new positives in their lives, and accountability for their self-care. Don't we all know that talking about their problems every session and never making change is keeping them from moving forward and healing themselves? It's up to us to help them discover what works for them and to help them move forward. We cannot legally counsel them, but if we are great listeners, we can help them discover for themselves what changes they can make on their own. Every session is about their process, and we can be an advocate for them to counteract their negative thoughts and habits by posing questions that they can answer themselves. A massage therapist who can help guide them properly to improve their lives—no matter what level they need to improve—should *never* feel afraid to lose clients to another practitioner. We want them to improve and transition to health and wellness and a positive health journey, right?

CREATE CONFIDENCE IN YOURSELF

Start with knowing the history of massage and what it was intended to provide. In 2700 BC, Chinese medicine led with natural medicine and treatment of illness. Shiatsu massage (acupressure) followed with the principle of acupuncture, using its own meridian pathways and assessment and using the application of the thumb as its treatment tool. Massage evolved through Egyptians with reflexology, and only royalty could take advantage of this. In the 1800s in Europe, Western medicine used Swedish massage, which was created by a Swedish doctor. In Sweden, doctors and nurses learned to administer massage therapy to patients to help them heal. Today's massage is based on Swedish massage and shiatsu massage. Please do your own research to learn how we have evolved in other time periods. It's a confirmation that we are medicine healers. Let this give you confidence when you are treating your clients.

Where this original intent was created is not what is provided in today's massage in a revolving-door-type clinic where a massage therapist is limited in how he or she can improve someone's life if the therapist is not actively involved in that person's care. Working for someone else doesn't allow a massage therapist the room to help a client in allowing the body, mind, and spirit to heal. Creating a plan for quality care for the client is our job; it may also be why we have landed in this line of work. If you think about it, we are a solution-based profession. Someone comes in with a need, and we are the vessel that takes that person from point A to point B. Having control of your own client base and being able to instruct those clients properly is taking them further, from point B to point C and beyond. By implementing this type of holistic care for all our clients, they will reach those goals. Without the opportunity for using this skill, how can we help someone accomplish a direction in better health and prevention of disease?

Note that when you are on your own, you are helping clients with more than a massage; you are helping them in their health journey. We have so much to offer them based on our skills, knowledge, and experiences, especially if we absolutely love what we do. We are more motivated to help people if we can see results in them. If that's your passion, never let it go! There is a reason you are passionate about it and why you must keep doing it. We have millions of people who need us to take the time to help them so a client who seems unhappy may leave your practice most likely because they aren't ready for the change. This should never be a concern if you are set up with a great referral system. If consumers have memberships to other places that have cheaper offerings, we should be happy for them since we know that sometimes choosing a cheaper massage is better than not getting a massage at all, particularly since we know that the therapist who works in the clinic on the corner has huge limitations of time in fully helping them. What we need to know is that this is not a threat to our business. If the clinic on the corner doesn't offer a proper plan for the client, we know that the client won't encounter any progress toward healing. This is why the independent practitioner is so vital to our industry—to carry out the results that massage was designed for.

LOSING CONTROL

For the first time ever I worked for a chiropractor for a year when a recession occurred in 2008. A word of caution: If you work for someone else, choose your health partners wisely. Here is my experience in losing control of providing the care I am an expert at providing. My household income was highly impacted, and I had to share with my two partners the payment for unrented space at a time when a lot of our clients collectively took massage out of their monthly budgets, leaving me with little income from the clients who were not impacted financially by the recession. I worked a ten-hour day and discovered I was limited in what advice I could share with the patients. What I noticed was that they took no stock in my advice. I had limits on what I could tell them, and they were following the advice of the professional they were paying, which was not me. It was strange psychology on the patients' part, but as the chiropractor set up their care, they saw only the chiropractor's viewpoint in accepting what he said they needed.

Clients will look to anyone as an expert if that person can first show how he or she can help them and be honest about what they need. In losing the ability to properly advise a client as the expert—as a professional in bodywork in that clinic—I saw how I could lose my skill in being able to guide the patients in the office the way I did in my private practice. I would have referred several of his patients to other professionals who could have helped them further. But since they were not my patients, I could not give them the best options. I earned money I needed, but when I saw how much money I could have made on my own, knowing what I know now, it really broke my heart and nearly ruined my hands.

We do what we need to do sometimes, but I could have saved my body and time making more in my own practice, even if I had been giving away massages for free with my gift certificate program. Additionally, I had to sign a noncompete agreement when I left, which I was happy to do since I realized these patients would never seek me out since their loyalty was to him, and since he offered convenience too. We see this all the time in clinics that hire massage therapists. If you are a therapist who has left such a place and had to sign a noncompete agreement as I did, you will be limited in your ability to gain clients, especially in a small town or area. This is destructive to the career of the therapist and makes it that much harder to restart and, more importantly, it makes it harder to start on your own if you worked for someone out of school. I lasted a year working for the chiropractor after I had been working for myself for thirteen years. I woke up one day and said there had to be a better way. Then I learned how to build a business out of my practice.

SUPPORT AND SUCCESS IN FINDING YOUR STYLE

Through our own experiences in business, you will learn what to do and what not to do. Now with social media, we have community with one another, and ultimately that brings us to a higher level, and we can have the confidence to be on our own. You can take advice from everyone, but don't follow advice that doesn't bring success for you. This advice can always be considered and dismissed and changed. While there is freedom in adding what does work or dropping what doesn't work, you must never waiver on the way to structuring your business to create success. Learn from others, but develop your massage and business style based on you, not someone else. It may take years to evolve into what you want to be if you are not open to learning more about business and new massage techniques to offer. Being able to recognize the body's processes is essential to your success. If you are an average massage therapist, you won't be successful with a massage business, so strive to be the best by learning what you can for you and your clients. Your clients should be able to do things again that they couldn't do prior to seeing you. They should be able to have a better outlook on life, notice the small things you have helped them achieve again, and be grateful to you for how you have helped them.

Your approach and style will evolve and change over many years, and this is great. You always want to have metamorphosis in your practice and be able to deliver results, whatever the changes might be. Trade with other professionals who have done this; learn from them in their successes and mistakes. A sense of community within our industry remains so crucial to our impact across the country. However, there is a lot of advice out there that is extreme and won't fit your style, so listen wisely and don't argue about it. We are all here to help one another; it's OK to be different. Use one another as support, and seek resources to continually better your desire to help others.

capturing your inner ceo

ONE OF THE HARDEST TRANSITIONS in our profession is taking everything we have learned in school and turning it into our practice. Until you start working on more bodies, it is hard to capture your own style. As soon as you exit school, you are focused on where you are going to land, where you can get clients, what kind of work you are going to do, and how to make money, right?

This is exactly how to get started, except that our dreams are often higher than reality. When we get out there and start working, fear can set in, and it can often be paralyzing. What was the reason you went to school in the first place? To work for yourself, to make more money than you were making, or to help others? Or all of it? If you chose to work for yourself, you have a big job to do, and that is to not only get off the ground running with your work but also make a plan for your business, how you will brand yourself, and what your niche market will be. If you are going out to help everyone, that is great. However, practice learning what you like and what you don't like. If you establish your practice focusing on helping everyone, you may be limiting yourself in how you can grow, and limiting your income in the process. Helping everyone can still be part of your business, but showing yourself as an expert in a niche market is what you will lead with to do this.

If you have concerns about starting your own practice right out of school, you are not alone—everyone experiences this. Why? Most schools are teaching you skills for basic clinic massage. They often do not provide information on how to create a business in massage therapy. They are providing a limited mind-set to students from the start, and most graduates go with what they are told. Many times students are going in with an expectation of working on their own, only to find out they won't get that in their education.

The fact is that everyone coming out of a comprehensive massage program of eight hundred hours or more is absolutely capable of working on his or her own and does *not* need "experience" to start his or her own practice. The word "practice" means just that—you practice your skills on clients, and you learn. You run a practice in which you see clients. Remember that we are not all masters out of school; we do need to have more work under our hands to refine our skills. This can easily be done on your own. The advice, "You need to gain experience before getting your own clients," is quite frankly—crap. This is the most irritatingly poor advice that I've heard over and over with new therapists. How is working for someone else getting you more experience? That advice is fear based, creating doubt in your mind about whether you can succeed. Your success is based on how you become your own CEO; most trade schools don't teach this skill. As you work for someone else, you are delaying the development of your style and yourself as a full-time provider.

Additionally, certain—but not all—schools have

their focus on numbers and their success with graduation rates. Some are designed to provide massage therapists to certain franchises since they are trained to provide the fifty-minute massage. This is an injustice to the enrolling student, who is unaware of the industry and the school's quality and goals. This has affected our industry in the most negative way. The mind-set is to fulfill the franchises' needs for business. What we need is a change in the demand of the market to demand better graduates. When we enroll in school, we have the desire to help others and trust that this might be a profession that we will love. The most successful massage therapy professionals have chosen massage as their second or third career, and this population of enrollees generally does better because they have work experience and because they have saved money on this chance that they can do something they might love to do. What massage schools have the ability to offer is an experience that is life changing. If you have been through a more comprehensive program, you know what this means. This is not comparable to education in cosmetology or other trades. Our education goes deeper and must be valued highly. Unfortunately, right now it's considered equal to other trade schools.

Others who are successful have someone in their household earning a second income or have a low-rent arrangement while they build up their client base. You have to be realistic to start out on your own. The failure rate for our industry is incredibly high since we haven't had the right advice, which includes the business training necessary to have a life-sustaining career.

For success in a massage therapy business, you must have the following:

- Business plan
- Referral system
- Tools that support your administrative processes
- Solid community support
- Coaching team when needed
- Mentor with ten-plus years' experience
- Business mind-set

A disadvantage that keeps independent therapists from starting out or staying on their own is lack of support; it can be a lonely profession if you keep yourself isolated. Sharing a room with someone or participating in a cohesive group of therapists who share space creates a fantastic work environment. You may have days where you never see one another, but you know someone is always there to bounce ideas off. These are people in your industry who help you make decisions and who you learn from. Learning from your own mistakes and the mistakes of others is a great way to improve.

Life challenges us when we really want something or make big commitments. The most disappointing thing is to see people struggle to make a successful income in our industry because of life situations. As caregivers, we can be influenced to be taken off track as we often put others' needs ahead of our own. However, to be a great bodywork provider, you absolutely must take care of your needs before anyone else's. Many natural-born caregivers are in codependent situations, and that's what makes them great caregivers—they are always on alert with a potential fight-or-flight response and can instantly serve the needs of others. We are here to serve. Now that you are professionally caring for other, you have to make your focus of having a business a first priority and the needs of everyone else your second priority. Granted, life can bring distractions, and for those who let distractions rule their future and cause unhappiness, their own life and work will always be a secondary priority.

Do you ever notice you draw a certain situation or person toward you who creates drama in your life? Do you have the ability to break the ties with this type of situation or person? If you can't or don't, you are putting yourself and your family second. Break these ties in whatever possible way you can—energetically, verbally, or physically. A great resource list of classes is in our resource section. Create the boundaries with a statement such as, "I have my business to run, so we will need to find some time to talk about this later." If you make yourself available, you will be sucked dry. It's your decision to continue on the path of distraction, and often distractions can make you stronger as you work harder for what you want. They are the roadblocks of life. Your job is to find out how to get around the roadblocks and find support to get through them. Roadblocks are usually brief, and the road can reopen on your watch in almost every case. When you change your mind-set on this and create healthy boundaries, you might catch some flak from your loved ones in expressing this new part of you. What you are doing here is creating your new self, the mind-set of you as a CEO. If you're sensitive, you may worry at first, but if you care about your path and making yourself a successful professional, this is one area of your life you will need to change to keep going forward and get what *you* want out of life. This is not selfish but self-care and self-preservation.

Here are some tips that will help you develop yourself as a business owner and help you and your company rise above other places that offer massage:

- First, you need to know why you are doing the work. This could be a journaling process that you have already started. Perhaps massage helped you, and you want others to have the same experience. Perhaps you have always had the desire and wanted to help people realize their health path. Or perhaps you feel great when you have your hands in healing. Know what really drives you to want to help others and do the work.

- Confidence! It's of utmost importance in starting a business and presenting yourself as an expert. You have the training that gets you started. That's great, but it's only the beginning of your work as a massage therapy professional. You absolutely must continue enhancing your skill set and refining the work that you do. If you are not learning more from continuing education, you are doing yourself and your clients a disservice. It is here that you build confidence in what you offer and what type of client you want to draw into your practice. Refining your skills is an absolute must in our profession, and it sets you apart from everyone. People will be drawn to you the more active you are in building yourself up as an expert, and that can only be done with continued hands-on learning. Taking courses online will limit your growth for interacting with other therapists, deter the expansion of your hands-on skills, and keep you in a box.

- Who are you, and why would someone—either a client or power partner—work with you? The story of your path leading you to massage school is a perfect beginning to your story. People must get to know who you are so they can help you build your business. It's often in our field that we do not like to talk about ourselves, but our experiences are valuable for others to learn, and our skills and what type of work we decide to do become part of that story. What they want to know is who you have worked with, what kinds of clients you have helped, and why you have chosen your niche market. Not only will that help them know you better, but it will also help you get more business. Look at some CEOs who came from nothing and have built million-dollar and Fortune 500 companies. There are a lot of them. They didn't get there alone, but their visions were clear, and their stories are striking. Feel the same way about your story.

- This leads to vision. What is your vision for you, your future, and what you can provide? Do you have other dreams of expanding your practice and incorporating a community of practitioners, or do you want to stay on your own and be able to be a comprehensive therapist? If you know what total wellness looks like, how can you give your clients great results? You will want to add your knowledge in nutrition, fitness, and other healing modalities that are powerful tools to help them in their health journey. This can help you provide a portfolio of services, and you don't need a degree or formal training. You can have your power partners lined up for that. With your partners, you will find a way that works for them and you that is financially and energetically agreeable for you and them in helping your clients. Explore what you can possibly tap into as an offering that people need, and find a way to offer it to them. This is visionary nature and what CEOs possess—an ability to see something that needs to happen. They make a plan, and they make it happen. You can too, with a clear vision of comprehensive care and how you can deliver that to your clients.

- Your goals. You need a *plan*! Every solid business plan states its goals clearly. Your plan will be written as any business plan is for any company. You have a clear representation of what your business looks like, what services are offered, what pricing looks like, and what expenses you will incur in starting up and then on a regular monthly basis. Sounds like a lot of work, doesn't it? Well, it's worth it since you will need this as a reality check on what you can afford to start up and what you can't. If you can't right now, you have the information to guide you in how to get what you want. Include future visions of what you want into your first business plan. When things are written, they have a higher chance of coming to fruition than if they just stay in your head. Add drawings, and write out the highest dreams you can think of, creating them no matter how big they are and regardless of the costs.

YOUR DREAMS BECOME PLANS

If you stay with what you know and become comfortable staying within that arena, and if what you have created is disconnected from your dreams, stop and reconnect with them. If you say to yourself, "I'm OK with where I'm at," have you thought of future plans for yourself or your family? How are you going to get there? The key to your success is to make something of your skill, become an expert, and use your expertise to guide others and teach others. And then create your retirement around that teaching.

Examples are to write a book, develop a training, and become a speaker and an educator. What you create now will set you up for life if you do it correctly.

honoring yourself

ONE OF THE KEY ELEMENTS TO A LONG career is maintaining a regular schedule—part of a weekly routine—of self-care in body, mind, and spirit. When you integrate yourself into receiving the work and processing emotions, you are feeding your journey of wellness while also learning new modalities of care you can integrate into client care. You are also shedding all the issues in your tissues to best serve your clients. Keeping yourself on one track of learning about bodywork limits your ability to provide more for the people you are trying to care for in your practice, and it also limits your potential to help people heal and can, over time, limit your ability to generate income. We graduate with a basic education, and it's up to us to educate ourselves further to become higher-qualified practitioners. This can be done through having our own experiences of emotional growth and receiving bodywork of all forms. It is through our self-care experiences that we become great practitioners because our education is enhanced as we understand how many different types of bodywork are out there and how we can expand our offerings to clients. Self-care is a mandatory practice that if ignored will create burnout. Caring for yourself allows you to take care of others.

Emotional growth and experiences with your clients will form you into the practitioner you hope to become. It is through life's experiences that we become who we are in our everyday life, and our clients who choose us—whether they produce a positive or negative experience—are meant to show us what we are on earth to learn. Who you are today will be someone who is part of your past tomorrow. Nothing shows you more how transformation looks than witnessing a child's development and seeing what forms that child as a person. If you look back at your childhood, you see that everything in your past has landed you in this career. You never fall into anything in your life without a purpose behind it. We are so lucky to be in this career, where we can express ourselves fully and facilitate the growth and development of clients, clients who are learning more about themselves in their time with us. As we provide an immense emotional safe space for our clients, we are subject to absorbing their emotional experiences, so we have to take care of ourselves first. Nothing will push you further in emotional growth than staying in this career, where your job is supporting your clients' emotional process and development, especially the joy they feel when issues become lifted.

Having your own practice may serve you better than working for someone else since you will have the time you need and can design your growth in learning more about bodywork and forms of healing. Often we can learn more about ourselves and our needs with more self-care practices. Any client's emotional release that takes place in your treatment space affects you in some form or another. An emotional release can be a scream, tears, sobbing, or a need to express emotion. That emotional release needs to leave their body to enhance healing. This can often be alarming at first, but supporting a client in the moment is valuable to that client. In this type of experience, you need to follow up with self-care to release your experience as well.

Over time, if you are not creating your own self-care, you will eventually have emotional burnout, and things will start to "happen to you." You will have challenges in life that will be hard to endure because you have no strength left for yourself. Your emotional self-care can come in the form of a guided retreat, a silent retreat, meditation, cutting ties with the dysfunction around you, journaling, tapping into your higher self and spiritual connection, self-healing workshops such as The Way Through Workshop, and of course, transformative bodywork.

Create a balance of your energy through Healing Touch, Reiki, and any form of energy healing. That healing will shed what you carry with you and reveal and strengthen you as a healer and practitioner. As a person who let life happen to her instead of creating it, I was one who didn't understand energy work. I didn't feel anything when I received it.

I just didn't get it until I took some training in it. It was my experience in learning that led me to feeling understanding and knowing how our energy fields are affected by everything around us. You might discover that knowing more about energy work and healing will enhance your desire to practice a long career. As we all improve ourselves, we raise the vibration of those around us.

Aligning yourself with other practitioners who are like-minded is also a form of self-care. Maintaining your practice will be difficult if you are sharing office space with someone with negative energy and emotion. A safe healing space is challenging to create in this environment. Your spiritual self and healing self will be stifled and continuously challenged.

This brings us to the always-spoken word in our lives called boundaries. Protecting your boundaries is a difficult concept for some to grasp as they start out in their careers. It's also one we must learn about in ethics classes over the course of our careers. Ethics classes allow us to check in on what we are doing in our daily practice. Some people who go to massage school may tend to be people who are missing boundaries in their lives. In our industry, there are caregivers by nature and codependents by experience. Codependency is defined as "an emotional and behavioral condition that affects an individual's ability to have a healthy, mutually satisfying relationship. It is also known as relationship addiction because people with codependency often form or maintain relationships that are one-sided, emotionally destructive and/or abusive."[3]

A person in a codependent environment at any stage of life will continue to draw those who need that person more than that person needs them. This happens in clients as well, so recognize if your clients are a mess and whether they drain you because they will need to find someone else. Don't be afraid to let clients go if they are draining you. Your emotional health is way too valuable to maintain. In my family history is some alcoholism with codependent caregiving. I have been conscious of the effects of codependency through relationships carried down to my generation. I was nearly going the same route and made terrible choices in my relationships. I had to break ties with this process. Part of it was done during my training at massage school, and part of it was done through counseling, which continued

[3]www.mentalhealthamerica.net/co-dependency

over the years as I attempted to find myself. For me, what worked was understanding that I was in control of shedding the person I thought I was through meditation, healing work such as Reiki and Healing Touch, psychic readings, and lots and lots of journaling. I had to shed my crap and shed the people in my life who did not have my best interests in mind. This, in turn, allowed my business to thrive with conscious intention, which was written and clear to me. I encourage you to continually write down your vision and goals and refine it over your years in practice. Recognize those things that may be holding you back—people, situations, and how you react. You can change all of these things; it is a choice. Establishing healthy boundaries—not only in life but with colleagues and most importantly clients—is essential to your success.

Whether you are codependent or not, your ability to create healthy boundaries is vital to your success as a practitioner, and it creates a happy practice. As we know, massage is intimate, and the massage therapist must maintain an environment of trust and safety. You are the one responsible for setting the tone and boundaries of your practice. Being comfortable with this is established over time and through your experiences. For legal reasons, the top things we must maintain are proper draping protocols, sanitary conditions, and clear boundaries that show your personal life is separated from your practice.

- If your client is your friend first, this is an exception in drawing clear boundaries. This person already knows about you and where you come from. If boundaries are clear, you can maintain this dual relationship.

- If you have a client who wants to know a lot about you, this is OK, but you must be discretionary in what you tell the client about your life. Keep it vague, and don't say too much. If you are struggling in your relationships, don't share this information. While we all want to portray that we are human and have our own struggles, we don't ever want to make the client's session about us.

- You are responsible for establishing the boundary of your relationships with your clients. Your clients love you for what you do and how great you make them feel. If they learn you are unhappy or in a bad situation, they may feel sorry for you or want to learn how they can help you. You can't have a solid client base if you don't maintain your professionalism.

- A client who wants to meet your family is a red flag. Satisfy clients' curiosity by talking about your family, but never let them into your life. You are a professional and need to keep professional lines consistent. Either keep your issues to yourself or take time away from your practice if your daily life is affected by your strained relationships. You owe it to yourself, and you owe it to them to stay neutral.

Self-care tools that may help are counseling, journaling, or a self-care retreat with a colleague or a friend or someone who is both of these in your life. Make sure this is a person who stays away from opinions and is there to listen while you talk without judgment. If the listener has suggestions for you to change things, and those suggestions are healthy for you, that is the kind of friend you need in your life. Just make sure your friends and colleagues can be trusted with your information and support you one hundred percent.

Another form of self-care is choosing the kinds of clients you want and letting go of those you don't want. When you have control over your kind of clients, such as your niche market or a variety of clients, it is the best feeling to know they have come to you for a reason. Never be attached to those who leave you since you may not be doing something wrong; it might be that it's just not the right connection. If you don't have the right connection with some of your clients, you will never be able to help them effectively. You want to help them evolve as you do; transforming their wellness journey comes from transforming your own. Accept the fact that you can't help everyone.

Break old patterns in your life, and this will over time let you see how you evolve in who is drawn to your practice. Attracting clients to you is your ultimate goal. If you are diligent about your own self-care clients needing self-care will be drawn to you. Self-care isn't defined only as receiving bodywork, though I highly recommend that you do receive it. It is self-love and selfishness in the way that you keep yourself to yourself. The word selfish can be positive too. If anyone challenges you about being selfish, just say, "I know how to love myself, and that is not selfish." They can't argue with that because it's about you, how you feel, and what you need.

marketing u

WHEN IT COMES TO MARKETING in massage therapy, the fact is we are in a business of people, so using online marketing and social media for our sole marketing efforts will take longer to establish a monetary return, and it will be uncertain. This is hard for an introvert to hear because as introverts we rarely want to put ourselves out there and say we are the best. Everyone needs to learn how to market his or her business. Creating marketing sounds like a great solution to getting clients, but the fact is it doesn't work the same for our industry as it does for other industries. Marketing for a massage therapist can take a long time if you don't know where to start. What works for someone else doesn't always work for you. Marketing is the process of interesting potential customers and clients in your products and/or services. The key word in this definition of marketing is "process." It involves researching, promoting, selling, and distributing your products or services. Advertising is attempting to influence the buying behavior of your customers or clients by providing a persuasive selling message about your products and/or services. Advertising is part of a strategic plan to maximize exposure to your business while marketing is accomplished through presenting and showing what your business offers. Advertising massage therapy is already out there, and the public is more aware than ever about what it is. Advertising massage therapy is already done for us so why would we spend money where we don't have to? In business, the goal of advertising is to attract new customers by defining the target market and reaching out to it with an effective ad campaign. Marketing is the method that works best for the independent business owner as the general public knows what massage therapy is and we have an audience that does not need to be persuaded to get massage. As an independent business owner, you need to focus on how to influence them to buy from *you*.

To begin your decision in what types of marketing you will use, you must understand what kind of marketer you are and what skills you need to be effective. If you are paying anyone for marketing currently, you need to look at your return on investment (ROI). What works in our industry is connecting with people through networking in small or large groups. People need to know who you are before they come to see you. Heart-centered people in business or in the health and wellness industries are who you always want to work with. In health and wellness, you will find professionals who care for their clients and have a common goal—helping people out of pain and helping them stay well. You also need to base your decision of whom to contact on what kind of client you are looking for. If you are in oncology massage, connecting with oncology clinics and with oncology professionals and oncology groups on Facebook is a good idea since those people and organizations will have interest in you if your messaging is clear. Go to the people who know your people.

When you don't know how marketing works, don't pretend to know. Hire a virtual assistant or someone with experience if you have the ability to put money into a marketing plan that involves a strategic plan to establish your web presence through search engine optimization (SEO). Your listing on Google must be within the first two pages to draw the consumer's eye, but optimally you want your business to be on page one to be noticed. Your marketing efforts will vary widely depending on your goals, and they will especially vary depending on your provider. There are many SEO companies out there; make sure the one you use is reputable, has excellent service ratings and a high success rate. We have one listed for you in our resource section. Your marketing plan will vary depending on your goals for your business. There are several other ways to accomplish this. If your goals for your practice are high in establishing a real business, you will use a different strategy than if you are working from a home practice. When you have certain costs to operate your business—such as rent for office space, internet service, and office supplies—your goals need to be higher, especially if you have grand visions for a future wellness center or medical clinic. If you have these grand visions, you need to plan to bust at the seams with clients and begin expanding. Have this be in mind for your goals, and it will happen if you have a plan.

A dream practice without a plan will stay a dream, whereas a dream with a written plan will come true. You can determine your pricing while being realistic about it in the context of the market, and that pricing will change over the course of your career. The strategy to make the most income is tied to what you offer clients in the form of programs and not in the form of the packages of massage sessions you offer. Clients are looking for help, and you have the tools to share with them. Have them make their goals with you so you can help them achieve them. This will show you are invested in their results. If you provide additional time with them, place value on it.

GOALS FOR YOU

What are your goals? If you plan to stay in the industry for a lifetime, your goals must have the potential for longevity. In this situation I suggest generating several sources of income within your practice that exclude outside sales; some of those could be residual income that brings profit to your business at the time and in the future. This could include teaching community education programs, becoming an author of a short or long book, offering massage courses, or teaching massage therapy education. Implement programs you customize for your clients and have those programs include monthly services and products to reach their goals. If providing massage is a temporary or part-time profession for you, then your goals need to be designed according to that level. For example, if you like seeing clients at a slow pace, then you wouldn't want to have large goals for them to attain. Meeting these goals for you is equally important—work more with multiple short-term goals for them and implement programs that match your efforts.

INCOME FOR YOU

You have to start with a plan for the gross income of your practice that includes what you need for your household. You might say, "I need a lot to bring home; I don't know how I can make that much." Your new statement must be, "I bring home $4,000 every month to support myself and my family." You no longer have to stick with a certain pricing structure based on what everyone else charges. As long as you provide excellent results to your clients you should be pricing your treatment plans at a higher level. Knowing your market is important as well. Your income is not your hourly rate. Your income is what you have in place that brings money into your business. You can create anything you want in your income, your practice, or your wellness center. Anything! We are in a prime market to capitalize on our industry and offer more to the public; they are looking for answers.

PLAN FOR YOU

If you don't have a business plan, you need to start one today. What you write in this plan needs to have emotion and a cause that would bring you happiness. So the focus now for you is to write and/or draw anything you wish for in yourself, your practice, lifestyle, and future life. Start with the household income you need along with any income beyond that for your future, develop your practice around it, and then we can talk about marketing. Why? How can you know what your market is unless you know what income you need to achieve? Your goals and your plan come first, power partners come second, marketing through social media comes third, and advertising, well, that's already done for you by the big box stores unless you are expanding your clinics. What is the income you need to bring to your household? Include what you want in the future so that when you move out of that apartment to a house, you have the income to sustain the payments, or when you need and want your next car, you can pay for it.

DETERMINING INCOME FOR YOU

According to a tax professional we had in our massage school business class the general rule to keep in mind for the money you bring into your practice is that after you pay taxes (about thirty percent of your gross) and expenses (twenty-five to thirty percent of your gross), you will have the remainder to bring home every month. There are probably many opinions on this approach.

Currently in our industry, we naturally determine our income by simple math calculations based on how many clients we need to make rent and pay other expenses. When we do this, we are asking the universe to keep us within those limits. Open up your determination to make more income outside of how many sessions you have. You are not defining enough income for yourself when your goal is asking for what you need and not what you want.

You have much more potential than you allow for because you're not reaching your potential due to negative patterns of working from "lack" rather than "abundance" or thinking that you need to stay within a certain range of price per hour. Is the price range in your area keeping you from making enough to survive? This is generally applicable in our industry because we are heart centered. As giving people, we focus on the happiness of others and helpful ways we can work with people, and we don't focus on our income, ourselves, and our own survival. What can you do today to elevate and recognize yourself as a business?

Perhaps you have been down the path of making a lot of money but found there is no satisfaction in the lifestyle that comes with it, and you settle into the massage industry standard rate, which averages seventy dollars per hour. Money may not be that important to you, but may need to be if you have dreams of being a worldwide philanthropist. If charity is your drive, then create a crazy amount of income for travel to help this charity or for money to donate to this charity. This is a cause in your business plan that you must not forget to include in your overall picture of your life and business. This is a key recognition in yourself and your relationship with money. Our industry has grown to have a price range per hour that is incredibly vast. What comes with that is a quality that is also incredibly vast. Spas have surpassed the standard cost of an hourly massage because they offer more than a massage. They have defined the "spa massage" as a massage with not a great deal of therapeutic expectation. There is nothing wrong with this. They have a business model to maintain, and they have defined their niche. Their profit and costs of services is based on an environment people are willing to pay for and products that are hard to resist. But now it's time to create your own business model to follow, your niche and own offering for your business.

FOR THE SOLE PROPRIETOR AND FUTURE WELLNESS CENTER OWNER

Let's say you have a goal of bringing home $3,000 per month.

- Depending on where you practice and your operating expenses, you need to bring into your practice $5,000 to $6,000 per month. Will marketing through a community newsletter, Facebook Ads, or local mailings be a good investment for you? The ROI on paper advertising if you choose to use it is very low unless you live in a small community and you are already well connected and well known. If your ad costs you $800 and you get one one-time client from that ad, it doesn't bring you the business that you need unless it drives repetitive business. How many repetitive clients does it take to earn your investment back? The fact is, you don't know, so you need to know how to retain them. Advertising doesn't do this for you; only you can retain the client to understand if the ROI is there. This is the most successful part of your advertisement campaign—*you*. Can you retain one hundred percent of clients that come through your door? Very few can.

- You need to invest in something that brings repetitive exposure. Facebook Ads, press releases, or a series of both can do this for you if they're done correctly. This would benefit you if you just wanted numbers of people to come in the door, and it would be more of a campaign that would lead you to spending more money when you came up for renewal. This is usually a fixed advertising campaign in which your information is advertised along with hundreds of other therapists and clinics through promotional vehicles such as Groupon or Spafinder. Neither have the capability to offer you a significant ROI unless you have the plan and the space to hire more therapists. Additionally, unless they drive clients to you in large numbers, their offers will never bring you profit long-term unless you have an incredible retention record and have your therapists sell programs and packages that bring you immediate income. You will make very little income from each advertising campaign sale because Groupon will take a large percentage of an already extremely discounted service. If you are an owner of a clinic and you have therapists on staff you need to establish a great environment for them. Therapists don't mind working hard if they have opportunity to make money, but if they don't get paid enough, they get burned out and become increasingly unsettled in selling you. They will leave you if you don't offer them a reason to stay. Giving them training on how to get clients and retain them would be worth your time. That would ensure that you could keep them busy and making a good income. You must have a good business model of profitability so you can pay them a decent wage. Fifty percent or more is the best rate to retain them. Otherwise, they will see that they are much better off going out on their own. Your profitability can be made more on other products and services within your clinic, not solely on the performance of your therapists.

- The most effective marketing is within *you*. The most successful therapists and those who work past five years in our industry stick to drawing in the quality—and not quantity—in clients. Your ability to express the following traits will bring you longevity and success.

Costs—Be willing to spend some money on your business, whether it be for ads on Facebook, through published ads, marketing on your website, scheduling software, QuickBooks online for bookkeeping and estimating taxes, supplies you need, equipment, business lunches and dinners, or books. There are many more expenses you can write off on your taxes. The most important item to spend your hard-earned money on is continuing education for personal and professional development. Don't be afraid to spend money, but be realistic about the chances of getting a good return on your investment for your business. Always have a goal of putting some of your profits back into your business.

Your image—Being able to express how you are viewed as a person and professional in business is vital to your success. Your therapy room must reflect who you are and be welcoming. Rules such as turning phones on silent and no vibration will be a welcome break to your clients. Create your staycation destination for them. Customize playlists for them. Does your branding express who you are and what you provide? Make sure you are meeting these requirements in yourself and in displaying it to others.

Your ability to present yourself well in person— How do you engage with people when they arrive? Make them feel like they are the only people in the world when you see them; make them feel special when they leave by walking them to the door. Show they are important to you by following up with them and showing how much you care about their well-being, even beyond their time in your office.

A defined niche—How you draw in the clients you want to work with is a highly important task you must achieve to be an effective provider. You might be surprised how well received your expertise is by everyone around you. They are willing to listen to everything you tell them, so make sure you are good at defining what you are looking for to build your clientele.

Goals and objectives for your success are clear and presentable—You have material to show them that displays what you offer and indicates that you have something for everyone, not only within your niche market but for anyone you want to work with. Your desire to help them achieve their goals will be clear to them. Have reference materials on hand to help them understand what your treatments accomplish.

A plan—Know where you are going and what you need to do to start gaining clients and then continuing to gain clients through power partners and through meeting new ones every week. You need a business plan, an action plan that accounts for your weekly action. It details your active marketing tasks, which mainly would be meeting with other health professionals and influential people in your community. Time is money, but more importantly in our business, *time is marketing*. Staying dedicated to a few hours per week dedicated to marketing time will bring you more time in front of people who can help you which in turn will bring you more clients. Have a structured week to build time into your weekly calendar and *do not* accept clients during this dedicated time.

Confidence—This is the most essential component in attracting clients to you. Confidence in yourself is noticed by others, even if you are not one-hundred percent confident in yourself. Perhaps you are not one-hundred percent confident in your work and the results you get. Don't let this stop you from knowing if you are referred to by your clients as the best. You are! And if you can't help everyone, that's OK. You know that you can help almost everyone you work with. If you can't help most of those you work with, you need more training. Don't let this discourage you. We are in a career of lifelong learning. Therefore, it's key to learn new methods and techniques to create longevity and more income. This will give you confidence and another tool to use in the programs you offer your clients, which in turn will bring you more income.

MARKETING YOU

Marketing yourself through *you* is time well spent. It's not taking time away from your office; it is looking for ROI of your time instead of dollars. The biggest mistake massage therapists make is not keeping set hours for themselves, their marketing efforts, and clients. This is where burnout begins. Compromising the time of these dedicated hours creates a longer road to success and reaching goals. Expand your goal to have a master retention plan. Rebooking is a skill that will bring you longevity in your marketing efforts. If a client is not ready to rebook, you need to tell that client why it's important to keep up with regular appointments. You know the reasons why that client needs to stay loyal to appointments. It's your job to share the benefits with him or her. You must show ownership in what you provide. If you are dedicated to providing the best to your client, you must also have dedication to yourself and your business. If you don't, you will not get the quality of client you are looking for—the client who makes massage part of his or her life. Instead, you will continue to attract one-time sessions or those customers who are look-ing for a deal and are not interested in being a client. You may wake up one day and wonder why you are not retaining them. It all comes down to you and the skills you have to keep them coming back.

WHAT'S YOUR PRIORITY?

1. You are your best marketer. You must estab-lish your efforts with power partners and clients. This is the number one thing to work on. I suggest using one to two hours a week establishing relationships where you have partners who want to help you, and you want to help them. Your power partners are those in your community—chiropractors, physical therapists, acupuncturists, fitness trainers, and nutritionists—who refer peo-ple they know and work with to see you for massage therapy. You can find these partners in networking opportunities and communi-ty events. Showing up in your community is helpful. Being your authentic self is your best tool.

2. Marketing efforts, such as social media and flyers, are a second form of marketing, and these efforts help you establish yourself as an expert. I suggest you spend five hours a week on consistent activity working on your online presence if you want to engage people to recognize your brand. Most clients are not active with your Facebook page, but don't let that stop you from creating activity there to attract people to your business. Facebook advertising works for some, but often your ROI is not recovered unless you pay for boosts and advertisements. A boost on Facebook is a paid service to allow your Facebook Ad to reach more people. Don't invest more than twenty-five dollars per boost.

3. Advertising campaigns require a lot of money that can yield little return and must be considered third in line in creating a strong business. If your business or wellness center is already established and you want to expand and duplicate that success at another location, include a team and a large budget in your plan to start a campaign. Your strategy is such that

you can calculate a positive ROI within a few years. Ultimately, it's your daily marketing efforts and not advertising campaigns that bring you success and will continue to drive business to you.

Marketing for your business is an essential part of growth planning and comes from a desire to help other people. Keep the focus on reaching more people and let go of the notion that you have competition. This must be a new mind-set in your daily life. Don't count on digital marketing to drive clients to you. While it's important to watch our competitors, it will only distract you from what marketing plan works best for you. While we want to help everyone with a massage, we cannot. Getting clients is like dating; it only works when both parties are committed.

When you begin to truly love yourself and your life, you gain confidence and begin to attract more people who see you are one-hundred percent available to help them in their wellness journey. Marketing is only part of an integral part of your plan for your business and supports you in your efforts to provide the goodness you have available to share with the world. Let a shining light continue to exude from all you provide. As you establish your business, it will constantly change and of course, so will you. That is the beauty and the reward that comes from being the massage therapy artists that we have been called to be and the strong business owners we are meant to be.

appendix i

THESE RESOURCES ARE PROVIDED to support you in your business endeavors, there are many more to be added and there are many that can be found online and more to be continually added through our accelerated digital age. These are the resources I recommend to you as you embark on your endeavors in owning your own massage therapy business. The more of us that see the rewards of entrepreneurship and capitalize on what is needed in our industry the higher the vibration of responsible care we will create bringing a higher healing level for all.

RESOURCES

Massage Practice Building, LLC
www.massagepracticebuilding.com
Your top resource to discover your career path in the massage industry, giving you options for starting out in business and ongoing support through Achieve Systems. Individual coaching available with Suzanne Eccher, LMT Author, Speaker and Coach for the massage therapy industry.

Achieve Systems
www.achievesystemspro.com
Top Level Business Resource and Coaching Program—Guides you through the process of developing a business at any level including learning how to build education and income streams to help you plan your future in the massage industry with Robert Raymond and Suzanne Eccher, LMT.

The 90 Day Success Express for Massage Therapists: A Proven System for Building a Client Base in Just 90 Days
massagepracticebuilding.com/books

BUSINESS RESOURCES

Firestarter SEO
firestarterseo.com/local-seo
Use code MPB

Business Networking International
bni.com

Paystri Credit Card Processing
paystri.com

Quickbooks Self Employed
quickbooks.intuit.com/self-employed

HEALING MODALITIES TO HELP YOU CONNECT

Healing Touch
Reiki
Feldenkrais
Cranial Sacral Therapy

WORKBOOK

Cutting the Ties that Bind
Phyllis Krystal
Found on Amazon and through
Energy Medicine Specialists
energymedicinespecialists.com

WORKSHOPS AND TRAININGS THAT ELEVATE YOU

Meditation

vacationofthemind.com/meditation-programs

The Way Through Workshop

thewaythrough.org

Discover Your Psychic Senses

soulburstacademy.com
For your complimentary webinar about how to tap
into your intuition contact Suzanne directly at
suzanne@massagepracticebuilding.com